ALZHEIMER'S

Life's

DARKEST

D I S E A S E

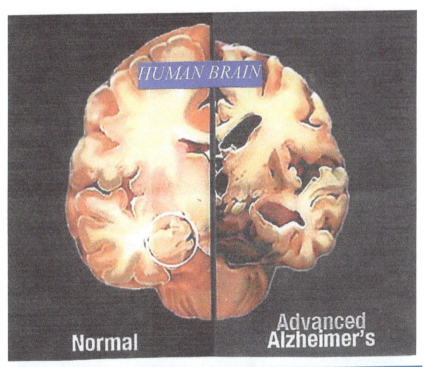

HUMAN BRAIN

Normal

Advanced
Alzheimer's

AUTHOR BILL BROKAW DESCRIBES HIS WIFE'S WALK INTO ALZHEIMER'S

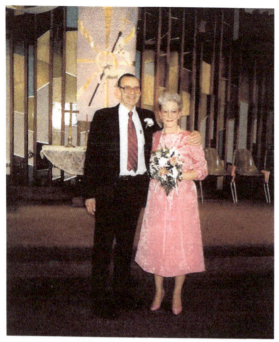

Bill & Pat's Wedding Day, May 30, 1992

ISBN 978-1-64515-337-5 (paperback)
ISBN 978-1-64515-338-2 (digital)

Christian Faith Publishing, Inc.
832 Park Avenue
Meadville, PA 16335
www.christianfaithpublishing.com

Printed in the United States of America

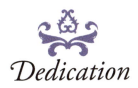

Dedication

*T*his book is dedicated to my wife, Pat, and to all those who are facing the future of full-time caregiving. There's no hard and fast guide to caregiving. One just has to become familiar with the behavior signs and take the necessary steps to understand what the Alzheimer's victim is experiencing. As I've watched my wife walk through the long, dark tunnel into darkness of Alzheimer's, I know she has gone through the anger of wondering why the good Lord has allowed this to happen. Finally, after many weeks of non-acceptance, she more-or-less accepted the disabilities caused by this disease. Extremely difficult for me as I witnessed her inability to do the tasks that she did so well before the early stages of Alzheimer's. As a seamstress, she had excelled, but Alzheimer's destroyed this ability. She kept trying, but suffered in silence as her mind and hand control wouldn't allow her to complete a sewing project. She was an expert at knitting, but that came to an end. She loved to monogram designs on T-shirts, but that came to an end. She continually asked me to purchase sewing supplies, yarn, patterns, and anything necessary to complete a project. I knew that none of these purchases would end in a finished product. Pat had great intentions, but did not accept the fact that Alzheimer's was the culprit behind her inability to complete a started project.

My dedication of this book to Pat is because of her determination to make a tremendous effort to overcome the pitfalls to this terrible disease. She fought like hell, but in the end, the clutches of this heart-breaking vulture made her the suffering victim. I do not know, nor does she, when the good Lord will take her out of the encompassing arms of Alzheimer's and into his arms of love.

3

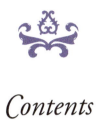

Contents

Pat Before Alzheimer's Took Over Her Life

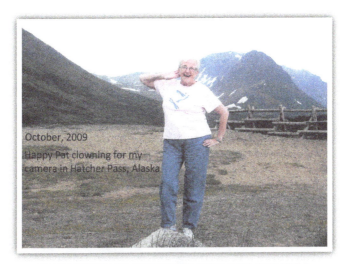

HAPPY PAT CLOWNING FOR MY CAMERA

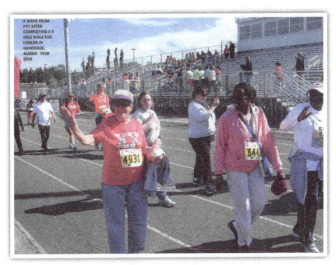

A WAVE FROM PAT AFTER COMPLETING
A 5 MILE WALK FOR CANCER IN
ANCHORAGE, ALASKA—YEAR 2010

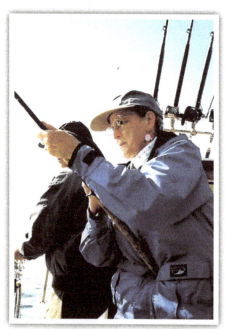

PAT HOLDING FISH POLE

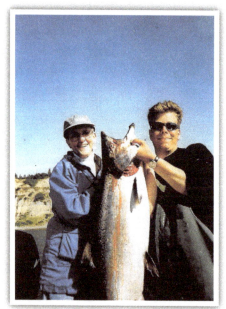

PAT'S HAPPY FISH CAUGHT SMILE

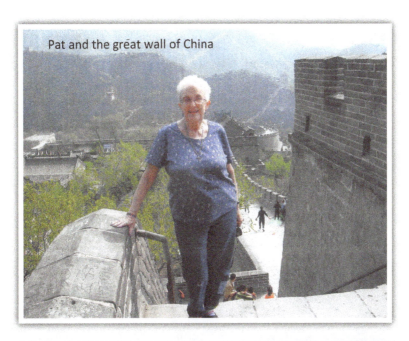

Pat and the great wall of China

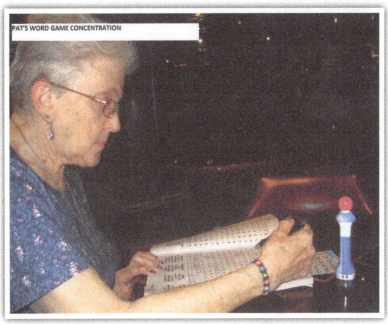

PAT'S WORD GAME CONCENTRATION

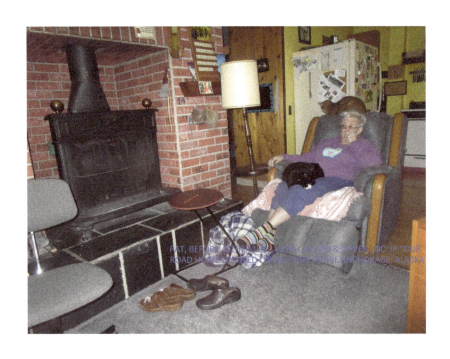

PAT, BEFORE ALZHEIMER'S, STILL RELAXED & HAPPY, IN OUR "OUR
ROAD HOME" LOCATED OFF ONE MILE ROAD ... ANCHORAGE, ALASKA

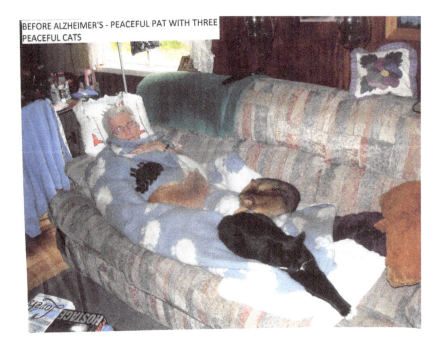

BEFORE ALZHEIMER'S - PEACEFUL PAT WITH THREE
PEACEFUL CATS

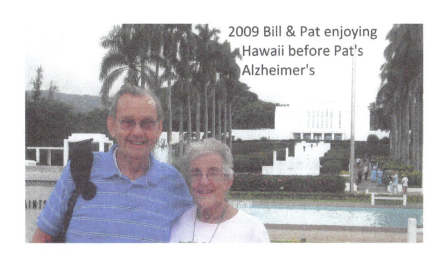

2009 Bill & Pat enjoying Hawaii before Pat's Alzheimer's

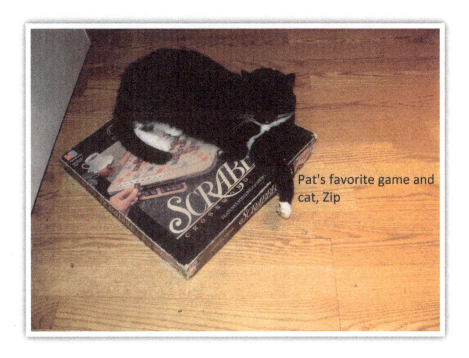

Pat's favorite game and cat, Zip

2010 Bill and Pat on Oregon coast beach
while enjoying Brokaw family reunion at Sunrise

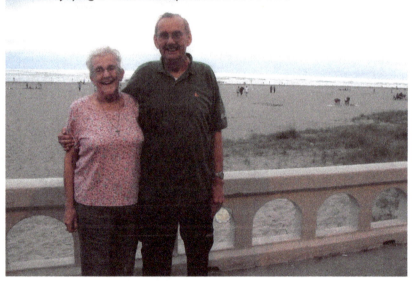

Chapter 1

As you begin reading this true story of my wife's walk into the sad world of Alzheimer's I would ask that you understand that each person undergoing this tragic walk is affected differently. By differently, I'm referring to the length of time the person's brain changes. Each person being affected by these changes has his or her own length of brain deterioration, and thus their ability to exist in the world of the uninfected is limited. The immediate cause of death is often a complicating condition, such as pneumonia, dehydration, infection, or malnutrition, but the actual cause of death is the dementia that is called Alzheimer's.

Since my retirement five years ago, I've spent almost four years observing and caring for my diseased wife. A job for which I was not prepared. A job that resulted in many sleepless nights of worry. I guess I didn't realize how self-centered my life had been before being forced into the life of a full-time caregiver.

At first, not understanding what Pat was experiencing, I became angry when she did not live up to my expectations. My friend Jan Gruhn, whose husband, Merlyn, had died of Alzheimer's, told me that I had to find a doctor who would diagnose Pat's condition. That doctor was Moe Hillstrand. I immediately made an appointment with her. Jan also thought that I should contact the Alzheimer's Association and ask for their help. I did what she suggested and found them to be extremely helpful in helping me to learn and understand what Pat was going through. I took many of their classes about being a necessary and understanding caregiver. Without their help I don't think I would have been able to understand Pat's disease. Sad, but it's a disease without a cure.

The purpose of sharing our story is to help others who may have friends or family members who are exhibiting periods of forgetfulness, memory loss, depression, lack of ability to focus, bedwetting, and bowel control. In my wife's case, these problems happened over a period of three and a half years and caused her life to deteriorate into a living hell. Lack of memory was a monumental problem and one that eliminated a lot of fun activities we enjoyed. The summation of these problems was the reason that VA Dr. Grant diagnosed her as being a victim of dementia.

The year was 2015 when I started writing what we both were experiencing as dementia entered our lives. Early on, I didn't put dates on what was happening as I didn't feel dates were important. However, in October of 2015, I realized that dates in my journal were important and would give readers an understanding of the speed at which her brain was experiencing change. I realize that what I'm writing pertains only to Pat, as others dealing with dementia or Alzheimer's may see brain changes happening at an entirely different speed. A friend of mine was a seventeen-year caregiver of his wife who was experiencing Alzheimer's. Another caregiver friend only had two years to care for her husband before death happened.

As I write this, I'm trying to use words that describe Pat's slow walk into the darkness of Alzheimer's. I do not know, nor does she, the length of this walk, but she knows what she is experiencing. As I watch her actions and try to understand her anger and frustration with living, I realized my knowledge of this disease was lacking.

She and I have been an important part of each other's lives for twenty-five years. The first two years involved dating, followed by twenty-three years of marriage. It was a second marriage for both of us. She had four children with her first husband, while my first wife and I had two kids. All our children are living normal, healthy lives. My two, and two of hers, live in Alaska, while her other two live in the Seattle area. Pat, my wife, has lived in Alaska for forty-two years, and I have lived in this state for fifty-six years.

We came together because of heavy involvement in our church. We are still involved in the church but not to the degree that we were at the time of our marriage. Pat and I help with communion serving. She is a lay leader, while I help with the collection of the offerings.

Our sexual intimacy was extremely strong during the first part of our marriage, but it came to an end about five years ago. As I think about this now, I think that it was extremely frustrating for both of us and something that we should have shared with a medical doctor.

In an effort to understand dementia and Alzheimer's disease, I have attended classes for caregivers at the Anchorage Alzheimer's Center. These classes have been extremely beneficial in helping me understand the severity of this disease and all the unknowns about causes and time frames. There's been a huge amount of research, but the bottom line is that causes are unknown and no cures possible at this time.

In October 2015, I decided to record the changes in her life as she lives with this disease. Pat was diagnosed by Dr. Hillstrand as experiencing dementia in its early stage. As I've accompanied Pat on her sessions with Dr. Hillstrand, I have become aware of what changes Pat has to initiate in her lifestyle to cope with dementia. Hopefully, if Pat can make the changes the doctor feels are extremely necessary, she will suffer less from the effects of dementia.

The number one change is her need to stop her alcohol intake. Pat, during the last three years, has found the need to make alcohol a bigger part of her life. I was aware of her increasing dependence on alcoholic drinks, but didn't give it much thought. She and I have attended one AA meeting, and the plans were to put the weekly meetings on our schedule. However, I'm uncomfortable attending these meetings as I'm a teetotaler, and Pat doesn't think she has a drinking problem. So I guess AA will not be on our go-to list. The alcohol has led to the second problem that Pat needs to change.

The second change involves a regular sleeping pattern. She is not to spend two or three hours playing games on the computer directly before going to bed. Computer games before bed is an addiction she couldn't seem to break. When she does retire early, I believe she returns to the computer after I'm asleep. While at the computer, she sips on some sort of alcohol. I sincerely believe that her alcohol drinking happens when I'm not in her presence. Her failure to get a good night's sleep and alcohol consumption have resulted in her need to sleep during the day. She will admit that lack of sleep leads to feelings of depression and despondency.

The time she rests during the day has increased considerably during the past year. Housecleaning is no longer on her agenda, although she does perform all laundry room functions and cooks some of the time. Her cooking is pretty much for herself, but at times, she will cook for both of us, but she relies on my food suggestion. She no longer attempts a balanced diet for herself, but she eats Chinese chicken with sweet-and-sour sauce, which she purchases at a local grocery store. I have to initiate our need for a healthier diet. She will no longer open a cookbook but will open a can or box of prepared food that just require heating. Following instructions in a cookbook seem to be most difficult. Recently, I requested a rhubarb pie, but she was extremely reluctant, so I performed the relatively easy task while she took a nap. An organized, neat, and clean home is pretty low on her priority list. I've always felt that housecleaning was the responsibility of my wife, especially when I was the working breadwinner. Now that I'm totally retired, and with my wife's dementia, I need to take over the chore of housecleaning. I feel she's very capable of doing a good job, but she doesn't seem to be able to organize the cleaning process. She's content not only to let me to do meal preparation but to clean the house as well.

At this time in our relationship, I realize my wife loves me but no longer wants to be responsible for meeting my needs. I'm not her caregiver at this time as she seems capable to care for her needs, but I do feel that her caring for herself is not the best for maintaining good health. She has not, and appears to have no interest in abstaining from alcohol consumption, developing a night-time sleeping pattern, and establishing a healthy diet. Her doctor had prescribed the above, but Pat has failed to follow doctor's orders. She does take her medicine for depression and dementia that her doctors have prescribed. Her doctor had also prescribed a regular daily exercise program. Pat does some walking around a school track, but that's the extent of her exercising.

At this time, I would say that Pat's experiencing the early stages of dementia or Alzheimer's, with time being the determining factor. I have observed her mental changes, but they have been so gradual that I have not been concerned until I realized that her memory, both short term and long term, has disappeared. Not only memory, but the inability to focus her mind on everyday living problems that need solutions. I feel that she has reverted to early childish thinking, which has resulted in conversation that is extremely repetitive and does not reflect much thought. It's hard to accept, but her good friends who have conversed with her over the years, no longer have any desire to listen to her childish chatter. Self-centeredness dominates her life. I believe her desire for acceptance results in much verbal expression which centers on herself. Seldom does she converse about the lives of others, both family and friends.

When she and I go out to eat or shop, Pat frequently initiates conversation with others by commenting on some aspect of their physical appearance. Comments involve others' hair, beard, jewelry, or attire. Once she receives a polite reply, she has no further questions but rather turns the conversation on herself, sharing information about her family and her life. She seems to thrive on positive comments from these total strangers. She has no concern about my need to wait while she talks.

Like all of us, as we age, our hearing and vision suffer. Pat was just barely able to pass the vision part of the driver's license renewal test. She has a hearing aid, but she has a difficult time remembering to wear it. I think her memory, vision, and hearing shortcomings are the result of the oncoming dementia. I think Pat is in good shape physically for her seventy-six-years of age, but the years have not been kind to her mentally. She has extreme difficulty focusing in on sitcoms. She always wants the television on, but she seldom has the attention span to watch and listen, and talks constantly during a program. She will join me watching news programs, but she will express anger when hearing and watching all the bad news. Soon after the news program begins, she will leave the room and transfer her attention to computer games. She and I both enjoy Scrabble, and we play several times during the week. Her ability to form words is fairly good, but she is impatient and quickly uses words that don't enhance her score.

I will share some of the behavioral incidents that she has experienced, that I have observed, and that indicate to me that she has dementia problems. I have been guilty of not realizing that dementia is a disease, and I have said and done things that have resulted in triggering her extreme anger at me and at herself.

The most recent incident was when she came to bed at 1:30 a.m. and awakened me with her body-bumping and constant chatter to one of our cats. At the time, I could smell alcohol on her breath. Needing sleep, I immediately moved to our downstairs bedroom. Sleep for me is usually in two-to-three-hour segments, so I was wide awake between three thirty and four when Pat came downstairs for a potty break, and then proceeded to turn on lights and sat at the computer. My presence surprised her as she thought I was still upstairs in our bedroom. When I told her that she needed to return to bed, she became extremely belligerent and angrily stomped up the stairs while uttering some profanity.

Another recent outburst came as a result of her driving to a nearby school running track for walking. I commented that it would be good for her, and that there was no need for a trip to the store. What should have been an hour or so experience, ended up lasting two and a half hours, and included shopping. I was extremely upset when she came home with stuff that were duplicates of what we already had and did not need. I told Pat this, and much anger and stomping was the result. I had planned to request she give me her Visa card, but before I could ask, she angrily gave it to me. At this time, I planned to keep her card in my possession. Upon observing the amount of money she had taken out of our checking account in the last few days, I had requested she quit withdrawing from our accounts, and that I would supply her with the needed cash. She has no interest in learning how I manage our finances, even though I have tried to help her learn. As long as she has money in her pocket, she's happy.

Yesterday, August 31, 2015, she and I had major food shopping to do at Walmart. We had made a list and were doing real well purchasing what was on this list. However, I became somewhat upset when Pat wanted to add an item which would have duplicated what we had at home. In the course of our rather heated discussion, she became livid and slammed her hand against a store fixture and angrily headed for the front of the store. After a request to return, which she ignored, I continued to shop. Eventually, after much searching, she found me, and there was no mention of her temper tantrum.

I will mention at this point that I have shared most of what I am writing with her two children who live in Alaska. They, in turn, have shared it with two siblings who live in the Seattle area. Because of very limited communication with their mother, they had no idea of the extent of their mother's dementia and were shocked when learning of her disease. One of her daughters, who lives in Seattle, immediately flew up to Anchorage to be with her mother. Her four children, now being aware of their mother's dementia, have set up a phone call schedule. So Pat should now receive a phone call each day from one of her kids. Her children have been very up front with her, informing her of the importance of making the life-living changes that Dr. Hillstrand recommended. I believe Pat is trying to make the changes needed, but is having difficulty. As I write this, she is resting on her recliner, trying to make up for missed sleep during the night. Sleep that is so critical to her well-being.

Repetition is constant in the questions she asks. I can sense feelings of fuzziness as she asks about days of the week over and over each day. Not only days of the week, but the activities we do each week. Our bingo-playing day at the senior center is the same each week, but she is constantly asking me which day we play bingo. Conversation, while playing bingo, will occasionally result in Pat becoming upset as she is very sensitive about her inability to remember answers to questions being asked. Sometimes she does not understand the humorous conversation of others, and her anger is very evident. Folks do not understand that this anger is the result of her dementia.

Yesterday, Sunday, September 13, 2015, I woke Pat at 8:15 a.m. so we could attend Sunday school and church. Waking is always very difficult for her, especially when she cannot sleep in till nine or ten. Sunday is a very important day for her, as she does enjoy both our Sunday school class and our church service. She does not like to fix breakfast, but she does eat the bacon that I fix, and does share it with two of our three cats. Dressing for church was not a problem, and she was always ready for the drive to church. Prior to leaving for church, I did ask her to make out a check for our giving, which she easily did. Yesterday, she was visibly upset when she found out the church women were having their own before-church class. Her memory had again failed her, as she did not remember that this meeting had been talked about the previous Sunday. The previous Sunday, she had also forgotten that she was to serve communion. Yesterday, she also forgot to wear her earrings and hearing aids. After arriving home from church, we each fixed a light lunch. Then, while Pat napped, I watched a baseball game and did some reading. I also phoned my brother and sister-in-law in Michigan. Pat shared some conversation on another phone.

After thinking about Pat's problems relating to memory loss, I guess I should mention things that Pat can still handle well. She is able to drive well, but I do wonder about her night driving. She handles her personal hygiene and is able to dress herself and take care of her clothes. Laundry is not a problem, and she keeps my clothes washed, ironed, and available. She is extremely proficient in knitting, beading, and Scrabble playing. She enjoys conversation with strangers when we shop or attend social activities. Bowling and bingo are activities which she really enjoys and handles both activities well. She really enjoys and appreciates the phone calls she receives from her four children.

Today, being October 8, 2015, I'll reflect on Pat's conduct this past week. I should mention that she turns seventy-seven tomorrow. Her birthday is extremely important to her and is a continuous subject of her conversation. Short bursts of anger came at church on Sunday, and Monday when she attended two church women's meetings. I think these resulted from well-meaning questions being asked by the women. I knew things had not gone well when she angrily told me she no longer was going to attend future meetings. Her anger was expressed at bowling because she could not remember which of the three games we were bowling. Also, she was angry when members of our team had to remind her to bowl. Sometimes she is more concerned with socializing than bowling.

I know she has been drinking alcohol in the evenings each day this past week, but I do not know the amounts. I found two unopened bottles of wine the other night and found them still unopened this morning. For some reason, they were left on the downstairs bed, which I moved to, after being awakened by Pat coming to bed after 1:00 a.m. Her alcohol drinking happens while she plays her computer games. Sleep is extremely slow coming after her nighttime sessions at the computer. She did tell me earlier this week that she is going to try to cut down on computer game-playing just prior to sleep attempt. She insists she is not dependent on alcohol, but I think she is not being truthful.

As I write this, she is lying on her recliner, located in our living room, and trying to make up for lack of nighttime sleep. Thankfully, I've been able to switch her from daytime TV program-watching to cable soft-music listening.

Today is Friday, October 9, 2015. It's Pat's seventy-seventh birthday. She worked at the Sullivan Arena from 3:30 p.m. until 10:00 p.m. doing her ticket scanning. A long day for her, as she has worked very little this fall. I decided to stay up with her until she went to bed. While she was on a potty break, I sipped the drink she had been drinking. I found it not to my liking as it burned as I consumed a small amount. Questioned her about it and she said it was wine. She seemed to be sweating as she was drinking while at the same time she was playing Scrabble on the computer. At 2:00 a.m. I was getting tired and felt sleep was much needed, but I didn't want to go to bed before Pat. Finally, I reminded Pat that she was not doing as her doctor had recommended, and not doing what she had told her family. I also told her I was keeping a log of her activity and was going to share this log with her family. She finally, without a comment, turned off her computer and went to bed. I know she was extremely unhappy when hearing what I had said.

Today is Monday, October 12, 2015. Yesterday, Pat and I attended Sunday school and church, after which we stopped and had lunch at one of our favorite restaurants. All went well at church, except Pat forgot that she was to help with the offering. Later at home, when Pat couldn't hear me, she realized that she needed to put her hearing aid on. She became extremely upset when she couldn't find it, and she couldn't remember where and when she had taken it off. We both have searched and searched, but to no avail, so will now check into a replacement.

Today, being Thursday, October 22, 2015, I will reflect on happenings this past week. Each night during this week, until last night, Pat had not slept well, and constantly complained of being tired. Her bowling scores have suffered because of her lack of sleep. Anger has been very evident because of her low scores. Anger, as evidenced by her pouting, and anger-triggered replies to others who verbally make light of her bad bowling. Last night, she had one glass of alcohol while bowling, but I do not know what she had after I went to bed. Attendance at a Monday evening church women's meeting caused her to be very upset when the one friend of hers dominated the meeting. She told me this was the last meeting she would attend. I knew that forgetting would not stop her from going to future meetings.

Chapter 2

*T*oday is Wednesday, November 4, 2015. The more I think about Pat's unhealthy eating, the more I think this may contribute to both her lack of energy and her constant need for sleep. Her dementia has taken away her ability to make good decisions regarding her need for healthy food, the necessity of a good sleep pattern, daily physical exercise, and the importance of water intake. I have created a form regarding her daily food and water consumption and have asked her to record what she eats and drinks on a daily basis. Hopefully, this will help her realize what changes she needs to make. I am going to use this same form in keeping track of my daily eating and drinking. So far this week, she has become angry regarding comments made by fellow bowlers, and while food shopping with me at the local supermarket. Her anger is expressed both verbally and through the need to physically hit something nearby, such as a chair or a wall, and she might throw something. Her anger is extremely short-lived, and she returns to her happy-appearing self within a couple minutes. If I try to question her later about her anger actions, I think the episodes have already disappeared from her memory. There's one older lady at bowling who is also experiencing dementia, and I think she understands Pat's dementia problems. She has been quite verbal with Pat, trying to help her deal with her dementia. Pat is not very receptive to her suggestions.

Last night, Pat worked at her part-time scanning ticket job at the Sullivan arena. When she had arranged her work schedule, she forgot about her Wednesday night bowling commitment. I bowled, but our team was short-handed because of Pat's work commitment. When she arrived home from her work, she talked solely about her work experience, with no question about my bowling. This lack of questioning is not like Pat before dementia.

Today is Tuesday, December 8, 2015. Pat and I had a good time bowling, with Pat having two games that were much-above her average scores. She had no anger periods and seemed to be her normal, happy self. After bowling, we both enjoyed lunch at Carl Jr.'s. We are now waiting to hear from the fellow who is installing a new driver's side window in her Pontiac. A week ago, she locked her keys in the car. To get into the car, she bought a hammer and destroyed the window. I believe this destruction was a result of dementia-type thinking.

This past weekend, Pat's daughter, who lives in Seattle, flew up to Anchorage to see her mother. She had been up here three months ago, and she wanted to see if Pat's dementia had deteriorated since her last visit. After chatting with Pat for a while, she told me that she definitely noticed that Pat's conversation reflected a deterioration in her ability to remember and think. Her daughter told me that she definitely felt that Pat should not accompany me on our planned twenty-eight-day tour of Australia and New Zealand this coming January.

My sister, who lives in Athens, Georgia, called me this morning. After hearing about Pat's behavior, she also told me that a cancellation of our trip would probably be wise. At this time, I plan to wait until January to make a decision regarding our trip. If I leave Pat home, I'll need a reliable person to be here for Pat, and I'm not sure who that would be.

Today is Wednesday, December 23, 2015. Normally, we would both be bowling in a Wednesday Night League. Each team in this league consists of five bowlers, which means there's a long wait between bowling, and this in turn causes our time spent at the bowling alley to be close to four hours. We both get tired, finding it an endurance experience, rather than being enjoyable. So I made the decision to cancel rather than endure. Pat expressed unhappiness, but said her last-night farewells to her bowling friends, and she said I was the culprit making the decision. We still have noon bowling on Tuesday, and Pat bowls at 10:00 a.m. on Friday.

Our Christmas, 2015 preparation has not gone well for Pat. In years past, she has bought Christmas cards, added short notes to them, and mailed them to family and friends. She has purchased some cards, but has failed to mail them. I have reminded her time and again, but she has made no effort. So there will be no cards sent from Pat this year. I'm unhappy about this, but have mentioned Pat's dementia in the many Christmas letters I have sent.

I'm having a very difficult time in my caregiver role. In the past, I have always allowed Pat her independence, but I now have to realize the importance of making her dependent on me. I know she dislikes losing her independence, but losing her memory, and her inability to focus on problems needing solutions forces me to relinquish her decision-making responsibility. I've had a very difficult time assuming this responsibility. She tells me I'm treating her as a small child, which is exactly what I have to do. Her thinking and conversation is slowly becoming that of a small child. Short-lived anger at my having to correct and control certain aspects of her life is prevalent. Her anger is usually expressed by stomping her feet, hitting an inanimate object, and throwing something she's holding. Anger expressed in this manner lasts a matter of minutes before she returns to her happy self. After these short-lived anger episodes, she is not receptive to discussions about possible causes and solutions.

Today is the last day of 2015. Thinking about this past year, I realize there has been a huge change in Pat's daily living pattern. These changes have to be attributed to dementia. Sleep and rest have become a very important part of Pat's daily life. Not sure what quality of sleep Pat experiences during the night, but I do know that she spends hours in her recliner during the day. Our laundry and the cleaning of our three cats' litter boxes are the two chores she handles without complaint. No longer does she make telephone calls to family and friends. These calls were extremely important to her in earlier life. Sending Christmas cards with notes to friends and family were always so important, but she sent none this year. There were always Christmas gifts and a card for myself, but none this year. I not only got my own gift but purchased gifts for Pat's side of our family.

Today is Friday, January 15, 2016. Pat's last day of bowling before we leave on our twenty-eight-day tour of

Australia/New Zealand. This past week, Pat has controlled her anger pretty much, except for an outbreak at bowling when she was unable to carry on a conversation with a lady who also has dementia. She was able to understand when I told her that the lady has dementia and was having a bad day. Pat is very excited about our trip to Australia/New Zealand and is sharing this information with the many folks she chats with, which includes bowling, church, and restaurant folks. Upon the completion of our meal in a restaurant, she stopped at one table and talked and talked, until I told her I would come back and pick her up when her conversation ended. She was not happy to hear this, but immediately stopped her conversation and joined me.

She still has sleeping problems because of the time she spends playing computer games prior to going to bed. She is taking over-the-counter pills to try and remedy this non-sleep problem. Her healthy eating is not happening, so I try to fix a little extra of what I fix for myself, hoping she will eat what I don't. We are eating more balanced meals at restaurants. Water drinking is still not happening, and Pat is always drinking diet soda or other similar drinks. She does enjoy beer and wine in the evening, and I know she has a tendency to drink more than she should.

Chapter 3

*T*oday, Thursday, January 21, 2016, is our departure day for Australia/New Zealand. Pat's having difficulty packing her bag. Have had to remind her of what she'll need for daily self-care. Also, I had to remind her about setting up a hair appointment. She told me of her need for a trip to the store today, but did not share with me what she planned to purchase. I shared with her that we have no purchase needs, but that I would accompany her on a walking trip around the mall. We did walk and window shop, but she became angry when I would not go to Walmart. I threatened to cancel our trip if she continued to have anger tantrums. She apologized, saying she did not want the trip canceled and would behave herself. I know there's much thinking fuzziness as she tries to comprehend the huge trip we are about to undertake.

Today is Sunday, March 20, 2016, and we've been back from our trip a month. Need to comment on Pat's behavior during our three-and-a-half week tour of Australia and New Zealand. The twenty hours of flying between Anchorage and Cairns, Australia, was probably harder on me than Pat. Lack of leg space was difficult to deal with, and lack of quality sleep was difficult for both of us. Being on planes for so long was extremely difficult for Pat as she was unable to converse with other passengers, except for very short conversations with those occupying the third seat in our three-seat section. Again, she had no interest in learning about others, but her only conversation interest is telling others about herself.

The hardest part of traveling with Pat was her constant need to converse with others, and her total disregard of the schedule we had to maintain. I constantly had to remind her of the need to be at a certain place at a certain time. She would merely look at me, nod, or respond that she would come when she was finished. I was embarrassed when she would tell folks about herself, and then tell them the same thing when she talked to them minutes or hours later. I told several of our traveling companions that dementia was the cause of this repetition.

Another major problem she had during this trip was bladder and bowel movement control. Peeing had to happen with little advance notice. Bowel movements were pretty much the same urgent need. More than once during our travels, she messed her pants, either urine or runny shit. This resulted in a huge need of a change of panties and slacks. Also, frequent showers were necessary. I had a very difficult time getting Pat to shower. I think regulating the temperature of the water caused difficulties. So I would take my shower and then regulate the water temperature for Pat's shower. Not only showers were difficult for Pat, but she wanted to wear the same clothes each day. We both took more clothes than needed, but only after my insistence would Pat change her clothes. Our very busy travel schedule made time for laundry almost impossible. We finally found a hotel that had an extremely small laundry room which we used. We came home with three suitcases filled with some extremely dirty laundry.

Finding our way around three of Australia's big cities did cause us problems. This necessary walking came when we left our hotel to find a restaurant for our evening meal. Fortunately, with the help of some folks in our traveling group, and total strangers, we were able to find our way back to the hotel.

Due to a problem with the strength of my blood thinner, I developed a swelling in my left leg that caused me lots of pain and the inability to walk without a cane. When returning from Australia, I had to be helped through both LAX and Seattle airports by an attendant who pushed me in a wheelchair. Pat was able to walk these long distances without any assistance. We survived this trip but feel future trips of this nature will not happen.

Today is Thursday, April 14, 2016. When talking to Pat a few minutes ago about her nightly problems, I found out something quite important. On Monday night, she went to bed at approximately 11:00 p.m. as I did. However, at approximately 2:00 a.m., I woke up and found her playing computer games and drinking alcohol. I knew by her conversation she was under the influence of the alcohol. Using language she could understand, I told her that she needed to be in bed. Her reaction to my request was anger. In her anger, she hits things with her hands, will throw things, and stomps as she walks up to the bedroom. At the same time, she is muttering how mean I am to her and that I no longer love her. I escorted her up to the bedroom and told her I would sit in a nearby rocking chair until she went to sleep. Took about forty-five minutes of her constant chatter, until her breathing indicated sleep. This same thing happened again last night; however, I only had to sit in the rocking chair about a half hour before she went to sleep.

Early this morning, while still in bed, I was thinking about Pat's nighttime drinking and anger at me for telling her she needed to be in bed. I decided I needed to ask her if she remembered what transpired in our nighttime, very anger-centered experiences. I asked her this while she was in a good mood and sitting at her nearby computer. I was quite shocked when she said that she had no memory of either of these nighttime confrontations. She gave me a very blank look and instantly changed the subject. Knowing that she is not always truthful, I think she may be lying about this, but I'm not sure. I do know that she is an extremely different woman during her dementia-filled days and her alcohol-drinking nights. At this time, she is back in her recliner, trying to make up for lack of night-time sleep.

In the early evening, two days ago, I was on the couch, while Pat was in her recliner, knitting. I knew Pat was drinking wine, so I asked her why she felt the need. She immediately became extremely defensive and was angered by my question. She grabbed her glass and emptied it in the sink and proceeded to throw something across the room, at the same time yelling at me about not understanding her, and how worthless she felt. She angrily swung her fists against the wall, threw something else, and stomped up the stairs. She also threw her glasses and some money she had in her pocket. At this point, not wanting her to do more damage to our house or to herself, I physically grabbed her and restrained her with my arms. I've never done this in our twenty-four years of marriage. I was angrily verbal and told her that she had to quit these temper tantrums, or she would have to go in a care facility. She, then, in her anger, put on her nightgown and laid in her bed. I waited by the bedroom door until she settled down and then moved to the downstairs living room. After a few minutes, I looked upstairs and saw that she had moved from her bed to her computer. A little later, she came downstairs and acted as though she had completely forgotten our confrontation. I'm not sure what the relationship is between dementia and alcoholism that causes Pat's destructive behavior.

On Wednesday, April 27, 2016, I escorted Pat to Dr. Mo Hillstrand's office for her scheduled appointment. Dr. Hillstrand started our discussion by directing her questions to me regarding Pat's performance since our last appointment several months ago. I was honest and informed her that Pat was not able to do what Dr. Hillstrand had recommended. Pat is still addicted to alcohol, to computer games immediately before bedtime, and does not have a regular pattern of sleep time. Again, she told Pat that her alcohol drinking was going to result in an early death. After much rather heated words about Pat's inability to change her lifestyle, she told Pat that she should no longer drive, and asked me to make certain she did not drive. Pat was extremely angered about this decision but did give me the keys to her car. Now it is up to me to drive Pat to doctor's appointments, events she enjoys, and to necessary shopping.

Today is Wednesday, May 11, 2016, and time for an update on Pat's behavior. She's having an extremely difficult time dealing with the doctors' demand that she stop driving. Now that I'm her chauffeur, she's constantly telling me where I need to take her for her shopping needs. Actually, they're not needs but wants. In my opinion, her wants are not significant to warrant a five-mile plus driving trip to a specialty store. She realizes I'm not happy about her constant requests, and she hopes I will relent and return her car keys so she can drive. But this is not going to happen. For her own safety, and the safety of others, it is necessary that her driving privilege be discontinued. It really angers her to not be driving. Every day she gripes about the doctors' request that she quit driving. After the decision, I constantly reminded her that her dementia was the reason and that our concern was for her safety and the safety of others.

Today is the seventeenth of June, 2016. She and I are going to attend an hour-long session at the Alzheimer's Resource Center. The session involves painting or coloring pictures by both caregivers and those experiencing some form of dementia. The hour-long session is led by trained dementia folks and is a very lighthearted, social hour with lots of humorous stories. Pat really enjoys this experience as she is good at painting or coloring pictures and enjoys conversation with others in this group.

Today, I was extremely pleased that she was willing to take a shower. There was no argument when I suggested her need for a shower. She did take her dementia and depression pills at my suggestion and checked quantities she has left.

This past week, she and I made a camping trip to Whittier. Spent one night, which was almost too much for Pat. As soon as we arrived there, she was ready and very vocal about going home. I fixed our meals while she visited other campers. Her constant conversation with me was about going home. Because of high winds, I did not fish nor ride my bike, but drove around beautiful Whittier and spent evening time playing Scrabble with Pat.

I have noticed that Pat is now using huge quantities of sugar. Not sure if this is a substitute for the alcohol she is not drinking. I have watched her put sugar in practically everything she consumes. Commented on this, but she had no reply. Checked with one of the dementia experts at Alzheimer's and she agreed with me that sugar was giving her a high, and was a substitute for her craving for alcohol. She suggested that Pat substitute Slender for sugar.

Today, June 19, 2016, is Father's Day. Pat would normally give me a Father's Day card and possibly a small gift. But this year, she merely mentioned that it was Father's Day and apologized for not giving a card. I have taken her shopping several times this week, and her small purchases have been for herself. This week Pat mentioned that our vacuum cleaner was not working. I took it apart and found it had not been emptied and the rubber belt was not working. We took the vacuum to a repair shop and found it would cost over $200 to have it repaired. While I talked to the repair person and a salesperson, Pat found other customers and clerks to chat with. So while she chatted, I purchased a new vacuum. She was very upset when I interrupted her conversations and told her it was time to leave. She had no interest in learning about my purchase. When we arrived home, she did vacuum our downstairs living area and was impressed with the vacuum's performance.

Wednesday, July 23, 2016. Pat's teeth have deteriorated to the point of the need for total replacement. The day before yesterday, Pat had all her teeth pulled. Three to five weeks are necessary for healing of the gums before replace-ment plates can be inserted. I have found Pat to be pretty amazing, as she has handled her teeth removal, and has only taken one pill for pain. She has dealt with the bruising dis-coloration very well, and merely laughed when looking in the mirror. I was quite surprised, that even though her face was badly discolored, she handled our weekly bingo outing quite well. She had no anger when folks were questioning her about her discolored face. She realized that folks were interested in the cause of her facial coloring and their ques-tions were meant to be humorous.

Recently, I have noticed quite a change in her daily liv-ing attitude. She no longer fights the changes brought on by dementia. She has pretty much accepted that dementia has brought huge changes to her life. She accepts, but does have a very depressive attitude. Her anger episodes are less frequent. She still resents me treating her as one needing my guidance. She has the feeling that I do not show sympa-thy, nor do I understand her dementia problems. She feels my role has changed from being her husband to being her father. Her daily repetitive questions are difficult for both of us, but necessary for her. I've had to learn to show gen-tleness and understanding when answering her questions regarding the day of the week and what's on our sched-ule. She is very demanding that we shop daily and have fun things on our schedule. Shopping with her causes me a great deal of frustration because she puts things in our shopping basket that we have at home or that we do not need. During yesterday's shopping at Walmart, I was able to take unneeded things out of the basket before we got to the cashier. Pat never missed them when we unpacked at home. I probably should write to Walmart apologizing for putting these unneeded items in the closest empty space.

Today is July 26, 2016. Pat had a night of restful sleep. I know she was playing computer games when I retired at approximately ten thirty last evening. I was awakened when she came up to bed at approximately twelve thirty. She came downstairs at eight thirty this morning but complained about getting up too early. She is now in her recliner, trying to catch up on missed sleep.

Yesterday, the two of us went to Walmart to purchase needed food supplies. We had a list of what was needed. Since I'm aware of Pat's tendency to pick up unneeded items, I tried to stay by her side. From previous trips, I knew that she would grab soda, something that we had an abundance of at home. When she did as I anticipated, I was quick to point out that it was a duplicate of what we had at home. Her anger was instant, and she threw the bottle with much force at the shelf, verbally accusing me of being her father. Verbally, in my anger, I told her it was best that we go to the check-out and pay for what was in our basket and finish shopping at a later time. Hearing my comment, she calmed down, saying that she would let me finish getting the items on our list. She did follow me, but I had to stop and wait while she chatted with other customers. I think her dementia causes these short-lived anger tantrums. I'm not sure how to handle future shopping trips. I know that shopping is all-important to Pat.

Pat is totally aware of her failing memory. I know that my memory is also failing, consequently, we're both in the same boat. However, it is my job to make certain all doctor's appointments and fun things we do are written down on a large calendar for both of us to see. I know Pat will not read, so I will have to remember for both of us.

Today is Thursday, September 15, 2016. I have been delinquent about recording Pat's condition since July 26, 2016. Much has happened during this time to complicate Pat's lifestyle. A train trip to the Alaska State Fair on Saturday, August 27, resulted in a major fall. Just after we boarded the train for the return trip to Anchorage, she missed a step and fell extremely hard, fracturing her hip bone. So besides dementia, hip pain, and dependency on a walker, life has not been easy for Pat. With Veteran's Administration help, we have obtained a walker. We received a VA doctor's diagnoses of the hip bone fracture. The VA also set us up for an appointment for further orthopedic help, enrollment in a daycare center, two hours, twice a week home-help for Pat, and ten physical therapy sessions. Although our military experience was short-lived and years ago, it is now paying big dividends with the available financial help of the VA. We feel so fortunate that we qualify for their assistance.

Pat's teeth, uppers and lowers, were finally put in two weeks ago. We were both extremely pleased with their appearance, and Pat said they caused her no discomfort. However, the following day, she complained of soreness when putting in the lower plate. So it was back to the dentist's office for an adjustment to the plate. Thumbs-up from Pat after the dental hygienist made some changes. So all was good as we departed the dentist's office. However, the next day, she complained again, but we decided to wait a few days before going back for adjustments. A couple days later, I noticed she was not wearing either plate. I looked in her plastic storage box and found only her lowers. She said she didn't have any idea where she had left her uppers. I thought I would be able to find her missing teeth, but several hours of searching proved unproductive. Pat's dementia and her inability to walk made searching a one-man job. Over the course of the last two days, I've spent much time searching, and at the same time cleaning.

While Pat attended adult daycare yesterday, I bicycled eight miles with two other members of our Senior Center Bicycle Club. Late in the afternoon, I was chatting with Pat about our day's activities. During our conversation, I was totally in shock when I noticed that Pat was wearing the missing upper dentures. Upon questioning her about the reappearance of these dentures, she was unable to remember or explain how these dentures happened to be back in her mouth. Dementia has caused a mystery that I'll never solve. I have asked Pat to make sure I'm around when she removes her dentures.

Today is Thursday, September 27, 2016. Reflecting on Pat's behavior the past few days, I find that I'm thinking about the need for Pat to be moved to a care center. I feel that she is purposely making my life a living hell. I'm not sure if her total forgetfulness is the result of dementia, or the result of her failure to understand the importance of self-care. Self-care, in that she will not eat healthy, even though healthy food is available. Her pattern of sleep in a twenty-four-hour day results in no regular hours, with nighttime sleep very difficult, and daytime sleep a hit-or-miss affair. She drinks very little water, and her liquid intake is primarily some type of soda, with or without sugar. Her primary exercise is limited because of her walker, but she is able to negotiate our stairs using her walker. Her conversation with family and friends has pretty much disappeared, but she does enjoy chatting with strangers when we go out to restaurants or sporting events. Maybe professional care folks at a care facility can help her to accept and experience good self-care. But, I'm not sure if her dementia will allow her to make these very important healthy, life decisions.

Lately, I've seen a definite decrease in Pat's zest for living. Her need for fun activities is definitely there; however, her enthusiasm is not what it was months ago. I think she finally realizes that her ability to remember things is getting worse, and that dementia or Alzheimer's is becoming a larger part of her life. Believe me, this is so hard for her to accept. Anger, that God has allowed this to happen, and anger at me for not doing something to destroy this terrible disease, dominate Pat's thoughts. Guess I need to be more sympathetic when I discuss what cannot be cured.

Today is Friday, September 23, 2016. Pat and I enjoy a one-hour time at the Anchorage Alzheimer's Center where Pat paints color-book pictures while I join others who are caregivers. Today I was asked to leave the caregivers and help Pat, who was vomiting in a wastebasket. This is something new in her life as I can't remember her ever having this sort of problem. I gave her some Pepto-Bismol and she is now sleeping peacefully in her recliner. Hopefully, this is not ongoing and something else that will complicate Pat's life.

Today is Saturday, November 12, 2016. The last three weeks have been hell, especially when Pat's anger at both herself and me has resulted in tantrums that have resulted in Pat's expression of physical rage. Her anger has resulted in stomping, slamming doors, and throwing objects. I do believe she is not able to accept the fact that dementia is a permanent part of her life. She feels that I do not know what she is experiencing, and that I do not understand the reasons for her outbursts. And that I do not love her anymore. I do admit that it is most difficult for me to condone her fits of anger and rage. My patience wears thin as I answer her repetitive questions all day long regarding days of the week, planned activities, and her need for shopping for things that are unneeded.

She did fry herself an egg this morning, and was able to eat it without putting in her dental plates. Since she usually sleeps until nine or ten, I usually have my six thirty to seven breakfast alone while reading the morning paper. While I was exercising at approximately 6:30 a.m., Pat got up, made coffee, and then proceeded to play games on the computer. She waited for me to get the paper and then took her favorite section and read while I fixed pancakes for our breakfast. Before I went to get the paper, she became very angry when I refused to have the television on. Something I said during breakfast triggered her anger again, and she threw something across the room and stomped up to her computer. I can't remember what I said. Her actions caused me to angrily suggest that I might have to have her committed to a care facility if her physical anger became a danger to both hers and my safety. Her reply to my suggestion was that I should just get rid of her! Again, I reminded her of her dementia, and that there was no cure, and that change was going to happen. And that I hated it as much as she did. She then calmed down and became her pleasant self.

Today is Sunday, November 17, 2016. The past two weeks have been extremely difficult for Pat and myself.

Difficulties develop when I leave Pat alone. She hates being left alone and is angry as I leave for church-related responsibilities. In her anger, she destroys something in our home. We have a four-sided wire rack upon which she displays the beaded necklaces she has made. A couple weeks ago, she took this rack apart and threw the beaded necklaces on the floor. When I question her, she just gives me a blank look and says she cannot remember. On another occasion, she lost one TV remote. I believe in her anger, caused by my absence, she either destroyed the remote or hid it. We have a touch lamp that we keep by our stairs. For some reason, in her anger, she destroyed the lamp and could not remember what happened. Today, while I drove to a nearby credit union for cash, she destroyed a four-foot glass shelf and some of the contents displayed. She was attempting to clean it up when I returned. She would not tell me what happened, but I knew she was very angry. I took over a very difficult clean-up operation, while she admitted nothing and enjoyed her computer games.

I now realize that Pat is a good actress, as she hides her dementia problems with angry words that she uses to make me feel guilty. She still expresses anger about not being able to drive, and she feels that I caused the doctor to tell her no driving. I've told her, that her destructiveness is going to force me to have her moved to a round-the-clock care center. She angrily tells me that I should do away with her. Then she would not be a burden to me. I have explained that dementia is an incurable disease and is something she will be living with the rest of her life, and that I almost suffer as much as she does. I married her for better and for worse, and this disease is definitely the worst. I will continue to try everything in my power to make dementia life as pleasant as possible for her.

At this time, I'm on the verge of locating a care facility, but first need to discuss this with her kids and mine. I'm really not certain at this time that her dementia is at a level that makes total hired care necessary. I do have long-term insurance, but I'm not sure how long the insurance would cover total care.

Recently, she and I attended a college basketball game at a local sports arena. Upon leaving the arena, I made a wrong turn and became lost. As I drove, in a panicked state of mind, I made what I knew were errors in safe driving. I hated to admit my errors to Pat, but she knew my feelings of panic. She said to me, "Now you know how I feel." Panic, confusion, and frustration are forever a big part of her life. These dementia-caused feelings have resulted in her being constantly *mad as hell* at life. She's still in some denial, but her hope for returned health is fading fast.

Today is Monday, December 12, 2016. As I think over Pat's behavior during the last few days, I realize that better care for her than what I can provide is something I need to plan for. Not only her inability to remember days of the week and the things that are planned for her and me, but she is having difficulty locating familiar things in our home that have been important to her life. Our bird cage, which I moved three or four weeks ago, is something that Pat covers up with towels at the end of each day. Yesterday, she told me that she was going to cover up the birds. I watched her as she started around the house looking for the cage. She finally returned to where I was sitting and said the cage, was missing. I pointed at the cage which was within four feet from where she was sitting. Wall light switches, which we are constantly turning on and off, are now difficult for her to locate. Her false teeth and hearing aids I had to search for yesterday, as she had no idea where she left them. I found them mixed in with her sewing stuff that is located next to her recliner. I have located containers for them and have set them on our kitchen table and asked that she no longer put her teeth and hearing aids any place else except in these containers.

Today is Monday, December 19, 2016. It has been a week since my last entry. During this past week, I was never so frustrated in my life than when Pat and I attended a UAA men's basketball game. Before departing our home, I had asked Pat to put both her hearing aids on and her teeth in her mouth. She told me she did; however, I failed to check her mouth before we left. During the game, I watched as she removed her hearing aids and put them along with her teeth in her purse. I told her part way through the last quarter of the game that we would not leave until we had both hearing aids and teeth in our hands. She immediately started searching her pockets and her purse and located all but her lower plate. She was extremely angry, especially when I searched and couldn't locate her lower plate. I was angered, too, and finally decided that maybe the lowers were at home. As soon as we arrived home, she found her lowers on a stand beside her recliner. I now realize that I have to check both her mouth and ears before we leave home, and will ask her to give them to me when she removes them.

Today is Friday, January 8, 2017. There's been no major changes since my December 19 entry. In fact, she's doing much better in keeping track of her dentures and hearing aids. One hearing aid had been lost for a few days but then magically appeared. Pat had no idea as to the location of the missing hearing aid, and how and when it suddenly appeared. I know these hearing aids are not allowing the hearing help she needs, so I have taken her to the VA for testing and new aids. She does have a buildup of wax in one ear, and this will be removed in about a week. New hearing aids will be available in about a month. I know that lack of hearing has caused Pat much frustration, and the constant need for requesting repetition.

Today is Thursday, January 19, 2017. After dropping Pat off at the daycare center where she goes for six hours, I purchased gas and then shopped at Sam's Club. Pat loves shopping and I don't, but it is necessary for our survival. The shopping experience, as we shop together, is miserable for both of us. We do make lists, but impulse overrides the list, so wants rather than needs end on the checkout counter. Pat's dementia kicks in full time when shopping, as lack of memory causes her to pick up stuff that we already have at home, or things that we definitely don't need. If our income was unlimited, I would allow her to buy what-ever she so desires. But it's not, so we have to be extremely frugal when shopping. We do credit-card shopping, so I am extremely vocal about saying no, while Pat becomes extremely angry when I say no.

Before dementia, Pat did practically all the shopping for our household needs, and she did a fine job. She prob-ably bought too much, but our working incomes were more than sufficient to take care of both needs and wants. However, limited retirement income forces frugality. As I drive us around town to the fun things that are so important and necessary to Pat, she constantly verbalizes her need to shop, and becomes agitated when I fail to stop. The fun things so important are bowling, bingo, sporting events, and church activities. She has real mixed emotions about her attendance at daycare. Something she doesn't talk about are other folks in her daycare group that are experiencing dementia and Alzheimer's. I think her inability to remember names and the activities the group experiences lead to her lack of daycare discussion. So I do not question her about daycare. I will add that I think she knows and understands the problems these folks are undergoing, but is embarrassed to talk about them. She will tell others that she has been diagnosed with light dementia.

Today is Wednesday, January 25, 2017. This morning, I showed Pat a Facebook photo of her daughter's family located in Seattle. Asked her if she remembered names, and she admitted that she didn't, and had no interest in knowing their names. What a change from previous years when she insisted she be allowed to fly down to Seattle and visit her daughter, son-in-law, and she especially wanted to see her young grandsons. Yesterday, when shopping at our local Fred Meyer's store, I had a conversation with a checker who had waited on us for years, and who Pat knew and talked about quite frequently. The checker asked about Pat, so I explained to her that I had left Pat at a daycare center before coming to shop. She then told me that she couldn't understand why Pat, in a recent shopping visit, had walked right by her without a greeting or even recognition. I explained to her that Alzheimer's had not only destroyed her memory, but made face and name recognition impossible.

Pat's most recent self-anger resulted in her destruction of a wooden folding chair. So many emotional problems that memory doesn't enable me to remember the details of conversation resulting in Pat's chair destruction. Her failure to wear her hearing aids resulted in my having to constantly repeat conversation in a high-volume voice. High-volume, which would be considered yelling to those with regular hearing. I think the volume of my voice must have triggered her anger, and thus, she stomped upstairs and threw herself down on a wooden folding chair with such force that she caused the support wood to splinter and made the chair useless. I was thankful she wasn't hurt, but had a hard time accepting her actions. She was angry when I questioned her destructiveness and proceeded into her bedroom, locking the door behind her. Her tantrum was short-lived, as she soon came out of the bedroom and acted as if nothing had happened.

Chapter 4

*T*oday is Monday, February 20, 2017. There's been no physical destruction of household items since the destruction of the chair. However, I think that Pat's thinking more and more about self-destruction. She seems to have lost all interest in healthy eating. She complains about the uncomfortable feeling when trying to use her dentures; thus, she avoids all food that involves using her teeth. She is unwilling to use denture adhesive to hold her dentures in place and dislikes wearing them. When she does wear them, she frequently has to take them out. Hopefully, her dental appointment next month will help with this problem. Her hip hurts, and her lack of energy is evident by her days spent in her recliner. I think her nighttime sleeping is much better, but her depression during the day results in extremely negative complaining.

Today is Wednesday, March 1, 2017. It's been a busy day, as I had to wake Pat up early (7:00 a.m.), as we had to make the half hour drive to the VA for additional blood work, a VA doctor's appointment with Dr. Lucy Curtis, and get a readout history of all Pat's medical work since we registered with the VA last August. I'm amazed at the amount of paperwork pertaining to all the VA medical help Pat has received. The paper, if lying flat, would probably measure more than an inch. I have to send this paperwork, plus a MetLife Long-Term Health Care application, to MetLife Long-Term Care Claims located in Lexington, Kentucky. A claim is necessary if I have to put Pat into a 24/7 care home. At this time, that would be a last resort, but may be necessary in the near future. Especially necessary, if Pat's anger at having dementia causes her to become self-destructive or Bill-destructive. Her and my safety are most important, and if she cannot control her anger and becomes a threat to our safety, a home with 24 hour supervision is necessary.

Dr. Curtis, with a student-learner present, spent an hour with us this morning. She was extremely thorough and had many questions for both Pat and myself. She didn't prescribe any additional drugs but would have done so if I felt they would help. She is going to consult with both Dr. Grant and with Liz Hunt, the director of senior services at the Day Break Senior Daycare Center where Pat goes two days a week (six hours each day). I think Dr. Curtis realizes that helping Pat handle her dementia is going to be a real challenge. She tested Pat with word memory and a test involving Pat's ability to put numbers on a clock's face and her ability to draw a cube. Both of these Pat did fairly well with, but word recall, day of the month, and the official building name was difficult for her. Dr. Curtis did not criticize or even inform her of her memory problem but continued on with questioning.

Today is Sunday, March 5, 2017. After much discussion about church attendance, Pat finally decided she would attend with me. This decision was extremely difficult for her, as she changed her mind about three times. Told me she would much prefer to go back to bed. I know sleep enables her to escape the realities of life. I told her that since she hadn't gone for the last three Sundays, folks were concerned about her absence. When thinking about this, I'm wondering why the women in our church are concerned about her, but not concerned enough to make a phone call.

Today is Monday, March 13, 2017. Pat must have had a sleepless night as it's now 10:30 a.m. and she's still in bed. I have things to do today, but they may have to wait until tomorrow, as Pat's sleep is more important. Every day, a crisis in Pat's life causes me to experience anger and total frustration. Yesterday, as we were preparing to meet her family for a restaurant breakfast before attending church, Pat was very upset about not being able to find her glasses. She could not remember where she took them off before bedtime. In prior instances, when she reported loss of her glasses, I knew immediately that they had fallen off the nightstand located by our bed, and I retrieved them from the floor. Not there yesterday, so I spent at least a half hour searching, while Pat dozed in her recliner. Not finding them, we left for our family breakfast. Since Pat was without glasses and had one defective hearing aid, I decided that the church visit would cause Pat frustration, so skipping church was necessary, and a trip home to find her glasses was more important. When we arrived home, Pat immediately found comfort in her recliner, while I racked my brain as to where to begin my search. What a wonderful surprise when Pat looked over at the junk and lamp-holding stand located beside her recliner and spotted her glasses. I immediately told her to call her kids and a friend and tell them the glasses had been found. Another daily crisis experienced and solved, but I know that every day will hold another crisis.

Pat's getting to the point where her desire for sleep dominates her existence. It's now 11:00 a.m., and she has not left her bed. We both went to bed at ten thirty, and after a short cuddle, which Pat demands, I went right to sleep. I did change beds at approximately 2:00 a.m. as our cats and Pat's closeness caused me sleeplessness. Just chatted with Pat about her night's sleep, and she has no memory of what happened during the night. She's already asked me about our plans for the day, and she has no memory of what I told her yesterday about my need for INR blood work and need to have our cars lights repaired. She might remember that I told her we might go bowling this afternoon.

I also plan to attend a women's college basketball game at our local arena this evening. While I watch the game, Pat will be drinking soda, eating M&Ms, and walking around the arena, conversing with many folks. Every person she sees, she shares about her cats, her family, her age, her military experience, and a little about me. Her dementia has been responsible for what I feel is excessive, mindless conversation. When she returns to her seat, she complains about the length of the game, her tiredness, being cold, and her strong desire to go home and lie on her recliner. I do forgo watching the end of the game so we can beat the crowd to the parking lot. I have to constantly check with her regarding the location of her teeth and hearing aids.

Today is Friday, the 24th of March 2017. Yesterday evening, Pat, myself, and a close friend went to the Anchorage Senior Center for bingo. Earlier in the day, Pat and I had gone to the VA center to pick up her new hearing aids. We arrived at the VA center about forty-five minutes before her scheduled appointment, so we went to the lab for some blood work that her VA doctor had authorized. Blood work accomplished quickly, but a half hour wait for the hearing aid doctor was necessary. Pat was very angry that waiting was necessary and complained constantly to me and any person who was in earshot. Even though I explained to her that we were early for our scheduled appointment, she still verbally expressed her anger. Dementia has caused her to lose her patience.

It's Saturday morning, the twenty-fifth, 2017, and Pat seemed to have a good night's sleep, and did sleep until 10:15 a.m. After a bathroom stop, she poured herself a glass of root beer and is now playing games on her desktop computer. She said she took her pills, but has yet to put in her dentures and hearing aids. Checked the bed and found that no bed-wetting had occurred during the night. There's no scheduled doctor appointments or activities, so we will only leave the house for a Barnes & Noble book pickup and the purchase of a few groceries. March Madness basketball watching is on my agenda. Pat will be playing computer games and asking me many times about the day of the week, and what we will be doing both today and tomorrow. A close female friend of ours called late this afternoon, asking how things were going. I talked with her first and told her about our days' activities, which involved picking up a book from Barnes & Noble and shopping at Fred Meyers. I turned the phone over to Pat. Pat became very angry, when the friend tried to tell her what she should and should not do. Pat felt like she was being treated as a child and angrily gave the phone back to me. I have told the friend before that she has to understand the consequences of Pat's dementia and converse with Pat as she would a five-year-old child, but with extreme patience and understanding. No harsh judgment should have been in her conversation with Pat.

After reading a book called *The 36-Hour Day*, I'm wondering if Pat's extreme depression resulting from having to suffer from total memory loss, can be treated with medication. Her anger, that she expresses to me and others, results from her feelings of stupidity, and she thinks that her stupidity is the reason for her memory loss. She knows she has been diagnosed with dementia, and she feels responsible. No amount of discussion about it being a disease that she could not prevent and cannot control with medication will change her mind. Questions about cause and cure do not have concrete answers at this time.

Yesterday, Sunday, April 2, 2017. A woman at church gave me some very simplistic puzzles that she thought Pat would enjoy. However, after putting them together myself, I felt they were so simple that I would only insult Pat's intelligence by suggesting she work on them. I will leave these puzzles where they are visible and see if Pat questions me about where they came from. I don't believe she will have any interest in working these puzzles. On second thought, I may be wrong.

Today is Monday, April 10, 2017. This past week has been a rather revealing week, as I spent an hour and a half with a good friend whose husband was a victim of Alzheimer's disease. This friend advised me to think seriously about putting Pat in a 24/7 care center. This would be more for my health than Pat's. It's something I definitely need to think about. Pat and I had a good visit with VA doctor, Lucy Curtis, who has prescribed new medication which she feels will help Pat have less anger, depression, and frustration. One of her scripts calls for half pills, so we had to go to Fred Meyers for a pill splinter. Pat takes these pills before bedtime. She forgot to take this pill, so I had to give her this pill and some water shortly after we went to bed.

Last evening, I had a serious talk with Pat about our good years together and about our dementia-caused need for major changes. I told her that I love her, but that this terrible disease was going to cause our living style to change dramatically. At this time, I don't feel a 24/7 care facility is the answer, but I do feel that she needs to spend more time at Day Break (daycare center). We're so fortunate that VA will pay the bill on this needed care. I need some additional time away from Pat, and she needs the activities that Day Break provides. After discussing this with Pat, I realized that she had not been able to focus on the changes I felt necessary. I asked her a very simple question regarding our conversation and saw total confusion on her face regarding her need to give me an answer. Her reaction has made me realize that life is pure confusion for her.

Today is Wednesday, April 19, 2017. Monday is now an additional day that Pat will spend at Day Break. I will take her to this care facility at 10:00 a.m. on Monday, Tuesday, and Thursday, and pick her up at 4:00 p.m. Was surprised, when I informed Pat of the additional day, and she had no comment. Her repetitive questions regarding daily activities are increasing considerably. I have all activities printed on a big calendar, but she would rather ask than read the calendar. Her lack of healthy eating is my big concern. Her primary diet consists of M&Ms, root beer, hot chocolate, no bean chili, one cup of coffee, and some soft foods that require little chewing. Restaurant eating is interesting as she drinks liquids, but most of the main course is taken home in a to-go box, and she seldom eats it.

Time really drags for her as she no longer knits, sews, reads, makes bead necklaces, or talks on the phone. She complains to me that there's nothing to do. I'm not sure if she enters into the activities at Day Break. When not at Day Break, her primary activity at home is computer games. She does enjoy playing Scrabble with me, but has a difficult time sitting in a chair for very long. Pat did amaze me yesterday when I watched as she played a computer word game. She was extremely quick in putting words together from a series of random letters. Probably much faster than I would be.

Today is Friday, April 21, 2017. Bingo-playing at the Anchorage Senior Center went really well for us last night. Pat did become very upset with me when I asked her not to remove her dentures. I was afraid she would lose them when she put them in her pocket or purse. She got over her anger when I said we could leave for home and not finish the bingo-playing evening. She did not remember that Thursday was bingo-playing, and she kept telling me that we were going bowling, which we did on Wednesday night.

This coming Monday morning, I will attend a class at the Alzheimer's Center called "Meaningful Activities and Purposeful Days." Hopefully, information at this class will give me ideas on how to make Pat's days more meaningful and purposeful. I know she gets extremely bored at home when she cannot do the many things she did before dementia.

I have scheduled a physical for Pat on Friday the twenty-eighth of this month with her primary care VA doctor, Dr. Grant. I will ask that Dr. Grant fill out a health history of Pat that is required if I have to put Pat in a 24/7 care center. I have application paperwork for the Pioneer Homes in Alaska, preferably the VA Pioneer Home located in Palmer, Alaska.

Today is Saturday, May 6, 2017. In the two and a half weeks since I last wrote, much has happened. The visit to Pat's primary care doctor, Dr. Grant, went well, and I think Dr. Grant is really trying to come up with the cause of Pat's lack of appetite. She expressed an opinion that loss of appetite could possibly be caused by a stomach disorder, so we now have a scheduled appointment with a stomach specialist in a couple of weeks. Dr. Grant also requested a urine analysis, which meant that Pat's urine for a twenty-four-hour period was put in a container and taken to the VA for analysis. This was done, and yesterday, I received a call from Dr. Grant who said that Pat's urine has been sent to Seattle for the analysis. She also mentioned that there was a calcium problem. She's still not able to say how these problems are related to Pat's dementia.

This past Sunday afternoon, Pat and I drove up to Palmer and checked out the VA Pioneer Home. A very nice facility, and one that either Pat or Pat and myself, may someday make use of. At this time, Pat's stage of dementia does not warrant putting her in such a care facility. But we do need to get on the inactive list. So, I've filled out the necessary paperwork and mailed it to Juneau. Waiting to hear from them. I need to know if the financial help from the VA will enable us to afford to live in this home. Also, I'm waiting to hear whether or not we will qualify for Medicaid financial assistance. We do know that my long-term care insurance will cover $70 a day for a 24/7 care facility. So, at this time, it's a waiting game.

Pat's failure to remember is getting worse, but she still has the ability to care for herself as to dressing, personal hygiene, and limited eating. She is able to fix herself simple food items such as soup, cocoa, soda drinks, and ice cream with root beer. Based on readings from her daycare center, she has lost five pounds in the last month.

Today is Wednesday, May 10, 2017. I have not seen much change since May 6. Games on the computer are Pat's major in-home activity. She frowns when I mention taking a shower, but she does, and does not have trouble with the taking-a-shower procedure. Last evening, when we were playing Scrabble, she could not get the score-keeping pen to work, so she threw it across the living room. I insisted that she go and pick it up before we continue on with the game. She really enjoys this game and has no trouble with the math involved in keeping score.

Chapter 5

*T*oday we will be visited by a care-coordinator who is contracted by our Medicaid long-term care office. Her visit is to evaluate the needs and care of Pat. Pat does not understand why this visit is necessary, and I also wonder why. We just finished the hour-and-a-half meeting with the woman representing Medicaid long-term health care. She had several pages of questions pertaining to both of us and wrote as we supplied the answers. These pages she will send to Medicaid, and they will have the up-to-date information pertaining to our lives as we experience Pat's dementia. Since we eventually will need to request financial assistance for 24/7 care, Medicaid will be asked to share in the financial care that will be necessary. Having this information now should enable Medicaid to give us financial assistance when necessary.

Today is Saturday, May 20, 2017. Had a discussion with Pat yesterday about our need to make a total lifestyle change. She listened somewhat, but was adamant about not talking about it. I realized the discussion of this need for a major change would only result in her experiencing anger, so I changed the subject, but not before telling her that my health was suffering from her attitude. She is extremely verbal and expresses many negative thoughts about her life. She has absolutely no interest in my activities and dwells on her needs and wants. At this time, I think short-term memory has left her completely, as she asks me over and over about things that we discussed earlier in the day. Sometime it involves things that we just talked about fifteen minutes earlier.

Today is Monday, May 22, 2017. I've decided to put in the required paperwork necessary for Pat to be switched from the inactive to active waiting list for admission to the Alaska Veterans & Pioneers Home, located in Palmer, Alaska. I called the Pioneer Home administrative office in Juneau to inform Gerry Butler that she should receive the paperwork this week. Gerry informed me that she had forty names on the waiting list, but because Pat is a veteran and a woman, she could be admitted sooner than many on this list. If Pat is accepted to live in this home, we have thirty days to move in. I am now waiting for a call from someone in the home's administration to tell me what the VA's financial help will be and what my costs will be. I have received a call from the Palmer Pioneer Home representative and was told that the VA financial help amounts to $45.79 per day. This amounts to over $1,300 per month. I have also sent additional paperwork to the Pioneer Home people in Juneau for another program that offers financial help to those who are in need. This financial need assistance won't be considered until after Pat is in residence at the home. I have no idea as to the amount of financial assistance that is available through this program.

Today is Saturday, May 20, 2017. Pat was visually upset yesterday when I told her that we had no fun things planned for the day. It being Memorial Day weekend, I feel the safest and best place to be is at home.

She received hearing aids from the VA yesterday. Was very satisfied with the help the VA doctor gave Pat in making sure the aids fit properly and selecting the right volume that Pat felt would work. Now I just have to make sure Pat wears them and does not lose them.

Pat is more and more dependent upon my help than before dementia. Finding her pills, finding things in the pantry, locating her teeth, using the microwave, and finding phone numbers, are a few things that cause her much frustration and in need of assistance. Her bladder control is a major problem and results in nightly bed-wetting and occasional daytime wetting. I have to insist that she wear her pull-ups and have pads on the bed that will make changing the sheets unnecessary. Until Pat can control her peeing, I'm hesitant about using our camper. Also, as much as I like to travel, both within Alaska and to the lower 48, I will refrain from planning any trips until Pat's dealing with dementia problems is more control. I know this decision will not sit well with Pat, as she is constantly talking about summer trips we should take. In the few trips we attempted last summer, she was constantly complaining about everything, and did not offer any help with preparation, cooking, and cleaning. It was definitely not a fun experience, and one that I will avoid this summer. I probably should sell our very nice camper. But if she goes into the Palmer Pioneer Home, I will be able to camp by myself or find somebody to accompany me.

Today is Sunday, June 4, 2017. This past Friday, I received a call from the VA Pioneer Home in Palmer. Was very surprised when I was told that a female room was available for Pat. I was asked if this was the time to move Pat into the home. I am sitting on the fence in answering this question. We are going to visit the home at one o'clock on Thursday, the fifteenth of this month, and meet with a social worker. On this visit, we will determine what level of care Pat needs, and if we really want to make this big move. We, plus a social worker and nurse supervisor from the home, will make this decision. However, the ramifications of this decision are huge. Most important is what to do with our present home and hillside property? I have contacted my son, and Pat's son, asking for help in making this decision. I know that Pat will be resistant to make this move. However, I do believe it is necessary for both my health and hers. Her dementia has resulted, not only in memory failure, but also has caused her not to eat properly. She now has real bladder control problems. Bedwetting is happening during the night, and constant sheet changing and washing are necessary.

Pat, After Alzheimer's Took Over Her Life

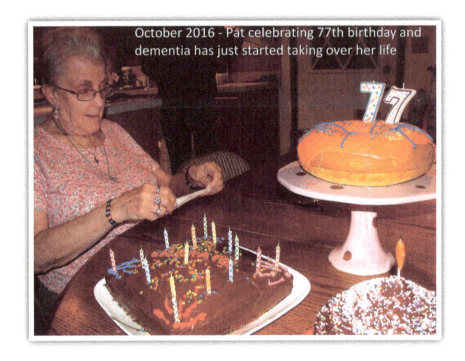

October 2016 - Pat celebrating 77th birthday and dementia has just started taking over her life

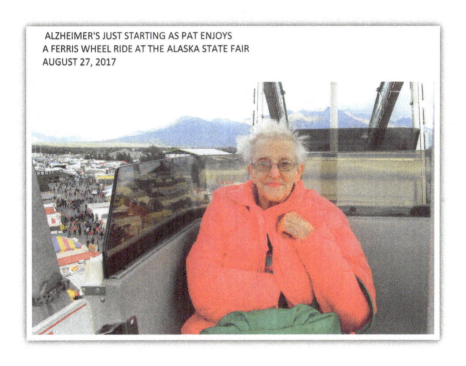

ALZHEIMER'S JUST STARTING AS PAT ENJOYS
A FERRIS WHEEL RIDE AT THE ALASKA STATE FAIR
AUGUST 27, 2017

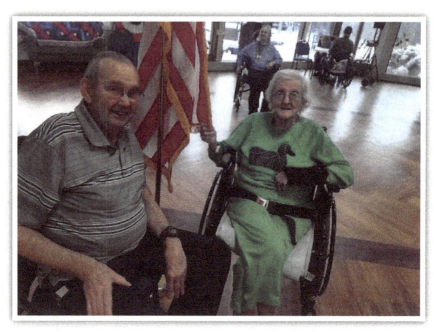

PIONEER HOME RESIDENTS REFLECT ON THEIR PAST

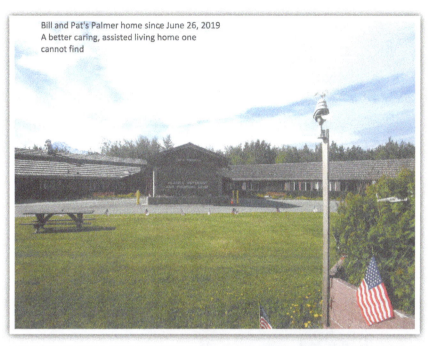

Bill and Pat's Palmer home since June 26, 2019
A better caring, assisted living home one
cannot find

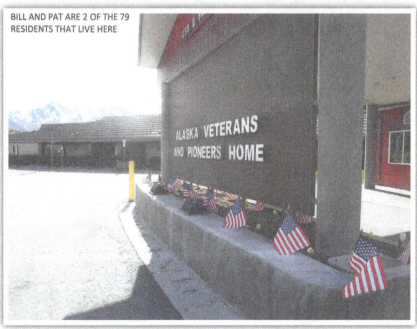

BILL AND PAT ARE 2 OF THE 79
RESIDENTS THAT LIVE HERE

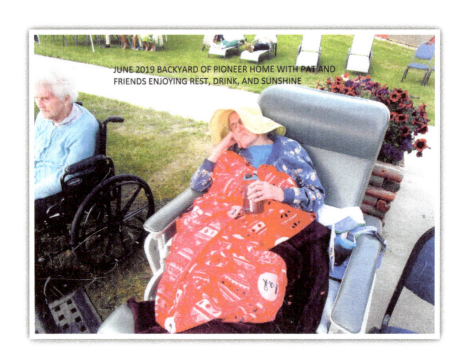

JUNE 2019 BACKYARD OF PIONEER HOME WITH PAT AND FRIENDS ENJOYING REST, DRINK, AND SUNSHINE

Today is Monday, June 5, 2017. Yesterday, in the early evening, after playing Scrabble with Pat, I told her I was either going to read or watch television. She became extremely agitated and stomped loudly as she angrily walked up the stairs to her computer. My hearing aids enabled me to hear her as she made some loud noise, before settling in to play games on our computer. Later, before joining her in our bed, I found that she had thrown the phone, causing the batteries to come out. She had also moved the fixture that holds our printer and the computer modem, causing a real mess that I cleaned up before joining her in bed. This morning, I asked her why she threw the phone and created quite a mess. She gave a blank look and said that she had no memory of these actions, and she quickly changed the subject.

She will not wear her new hearing aids at home, so I have to practically yell to make her hear. She gets angry when I raise my voice to a level that will allow her to hear. Because of her actions, I think it is definitely time to move her into the VA Palmer Pioneer Home. I will plan to move to Palmer myself, where I can be close by to help care for her. Many decisions, as we contemplate this move, especially as I've lived in this house fifty-six years. If I decide that renting is necessary, many decisions are necessary in deciding what to leave for renters and what we can find space for in our downsizing to Palmer. If we find the Palmer living is unsatisfactory, we'll return to Our Road. So we have to think about that possibility.

Before our meeting with the social worker and nurse supervisor at the Palmer Pioneer Home on this coming Thursday, I will make a list of questions that we need answered. The first question is: Since I plan to be of assistance in helping Pat, at what level will the Pioneer Home take her as a resident? And what help is available to pay the costs of this level and the procedure for paying? How many cats can Pat have in her room? What can we bring from our present home to put in Pat's room? Next, what arrangements do we need to make to have Pat's medications available? Is there a resident doctor who is available for immediate care? Also, I would like to know what activities the home schedules for their residents? Also, can I receive any assistance in locating a place to live in Palmer?

Chapter 6

Today is Tuesday, June 20, 2017. After our meeting with the social worker and RN supervisor of the VA Palmer Pioneer Home last Thursday, we have to decide if the room available for Pat is the answer. They have told us that they would take Pat on the level three, which is total care. However, they have also told us that cost would be $5,400 per month. Tomorrow the social worker will call for my decision. Much as I would like to see Pat in this care facility, I cannot pay the monthly cost of $5,400. When called tomorrow, I will have to tell them to put Pat back on the inactive list. This means I cannot transfer her back to the active list for six months. In the meantime, I will investigate what financial help I can receive through the Medicaid waiver program and the Pioneer Home Payment Assistance program. All the paperwork involved in these two programs will require four to six months of waiting and hoping. This long wait is not fair to Pat and myself, but waiting is necessary if we want the care that both Pat and I need. Not sure if we'll be able to survive six months at the rate Pat's Alzheimer's is taking her down life's darkest disease trail. Her attitude changes so rapidly that I have to be prepared to deal with both her highs and lows. Anger and physical venting come and go, depending on her reaction to my helpful suggestions. She knows I'm there to help her, but dislikes having to do what I suggest. I think, that because of her inability to finish sewing projects, she becomes angry at herself. She has started many sewing projects, but nothing has been completed.

Today is Tuesday, July 11, 2017. I still do not feel Pat is at the stage where she needs 24/7 care at the third level. Her number one need is for someone, such as myself, to be with her around the clock. Her around-the-clock care deals with her needs not wants. Being safe and away from harm is most important. Taking her medications and having food available is necessary. Making certain clean beds are available for good sleep. Making sure her bills are paid and handling bills that are necessary for living in this expensive world.

Yesterday, a call from the VA informed me that the VA would pay for an additional day at the day-care center, and additional hours of home care, but would not provide total home health care for Pat. Consequently, I will wait and see if Pat qualifies for Medicaid Waiver coverage.

I have received a letter from my long-term health care insurance company, MetLife, informing me that, based on their research, my wife is not suffering from severe cognitive impairment at this time, and that she is not eligible for financial benefits. I have replied to them, telling them that I feel they are wrong, and appealed their decision. I am now awaiting a reply to my letter.

I have received a call from Angie White, a MetLife long-term care specialist. She had several questions concerning the appeal I filed. She indicated she would do further research into our situation based on my answers to her questions. She indicated that I should receive a return call regarding the outcome of her investigation.

Today is Friday, August 25, 2017. Still no call from the long-term care gal working at MetLife regarding my claim for payment of some medical bills.

Today is Thursday, September 14, 2017. At this time, I think Pat is doing better than she was a month ago. There are still lots of questions, like, "What are we doing tomorrow and what time do we need to leave?" But she is not showing anger-actions like a month ago, and she realizes that her tantrums do not help. She still has a bedwetting problem, but does not mention it to me, but she does help me change the bedding when I ask. She is extremely conversational when we bowl, play bingo, go to church, go to sporting events, and visit restaurants. She begins conversations by commenting on others' clothes or hair, but quickly turns the conversation to herself or about me.

Today is Friday, September 22, 2017. This past week, the supervisor from daycare called me and said Pat was doing much better in handling her anger problems. At least on Thursday. Pat's always happy to see me when I pick her up, but shares little with me about what happened during the day. She asks how my day was. She's always eager to get home, and she immediately visits her desktop computer for games. After a few minutes at the computer, she's back downstairs for liquid refreshment and perhaps a dish of ice cream.

The day before yesterday, she misplaced her teeth, so no dentures for wearing yesterday. Hopefully, she'll find them today. I have searched to no avail. This morning, I was shocked to see a pair of hearing aids on the bathroom counter. This pair Pat had misplaced long ago, and she had received another pair from the VA. Now she has three hearing aids plus a pair we had purchased from Sam's a couple years ago. Because of the size, it's easy to understand why they come and go.

At this time, I'm trying to arrange for a trip for me from Anchorage to Lansing, Michigan. I have decided that such a trip would cause too many problems for Pat, especially because of her bedwetting and her inability to get good sleep. The VA will pay for 170 hours of live-in care for Pat while I'm gone. I just have to find an agency that will handle this 24/7 care.

Today is Friday, September 29. I have located the agency that will handle Pat's 24/7 in-home care needs while I'm gone to Michigan for the week, beginning October 18. Today, at 2:00 p.m., we are meeting with Ruth, the respite worker from Midnight Sun Home Care, who will make our home her home during my absence.

Today is Monday, October 9, 2017. Pat's seventy-ninth birthday. The meeting on the 29th with Ruth went well. On October 16, Ruth will bring the caregiver to our house for a meet-and-greet time. Then late in the day on the seventeenth, the caregiver will move in for her week with Pat, while I'm back in Michigan seeing family and friends. Pat is not happy about my trip without her and has verbally expressed these feelings. However, deep down, I believe she realizes that her comfort area is our home, and that travel would cause her to be uncomfortable. Her memory and focusing abilities have left her.

Lately, she has gravitated to me more and more and is insisting on knowing where I am at all times. She does have difficulty locating storage areas within our home of such things as toilet paper, paper towels, and food items. Physically, she is fine, making many trips up and down our stairs, but Her anger about her memory difficulties surfaces occasionally, but is very short-lived; however, anger does result in stomping loudly, slamming doors, and throwing small items. She will eventually pick up what she throws.

Today is Sunday, October 29, 2017. Since my return from a week in Michigan last Tuesday, Pat is having more short periods of anger-actions. She was extremely glad to see me come home, but she never shared with me about things that happened while I was gone. I think her lack of memory made this impossible. Her temper tantrums are getting more frequent, and stomping, swinging her arms, slamming doors, and throwing small objects accompany her anger. Heard from the supervisor of her daycare center about her behavior there and how disruptive it was to their other clients. Plan to talk to the VA social worker and arrange for an appointment with her VA doctor. Hopefully, there's medication that can help with her anger-actions.

The VA doctor did prescribe new medication, but so far, I have not seen improvement in her anger-actions. Today is Sunday, November 19, 2017, and church is on our schedule, followed by lunch with Pat's daughter, son-in-law, and son. Her anger-actions are much more prevalent and causing me to lose patience. I have to constantly remind myself that she exists in a very frustrating world, and that the culprit, dementia, has taken control of her life completely. The daycare facility (Day Break) that Pat spends six hours a day, four days a week in, is going out of business as of December 31st. It is extremely difficult for me as I see the anger that Pat expresses each day when I drop her off. When I pick her up, she verbalizes her joy at seeing me and talks continuously about plans for the evening and the next day.

Today is Friday, December 28, 2017. I still have received no word as to which daycare facility in Anchorage the VA will approve for care for Pat. I feel she, as well as myself, does need this daycare experience. It provides a place for her to interact with others and escape the confinement of our home. She gets bored easily and is always asking me what fun things we are going to do. She is not happy when I drop her off at the daycare center, but is extremely happy to see me six hours later.

Today is Sunday, December 30, 2017. Pat likes the thought of Christmas coming, but has no interest in the preparation involved, as she experienced before dementia. She has not done any shopping or even asked about it. Nor has she sent out Christmas cards. This was extremely important in her earlier life. In the past, she has always been excited about receiving Christmas cards, but now she doesn't even look at them when I leave them on our kitchen table. I am glad that she does attend church with me, even though her lack of hearing does not allow her to hear the sermon. She does have new hearing aids coming any day now. They are ones that the VA is supplying. I know she'll probably lose them shortly after she receives them.

Today is Tuesday, the day after Christmas. Pat is totally confused this morning. She feels it's evening and has forgotten that she is going to daycare this morning. We went to bed early last night as I didn't want to deal with her constant trips up and down our stairs. Steps that took her to the computer, the fridge, the television, and her bed. She has lots of energy, and the ability to use the stairs is not a problem. She had wet the bed and had changed her panties before going to the computer for game-playing. She turned on our overhead bedroom light to see if I was in bed. She then got a blanket and covered the area in the bed where she had wetted it and crawled in.

Today is Thursday, December 28. It's Pat's last day at Day Break care center. I'll be interested if they tell her that she won't be coming back. Yesterday, while she was at the center, I visited another daycare center called Hearts and Hands, and have submitted the necessary paperwork to have Pat attend this center. Hopefully, next week, she'll be able to attend this center. The location of the daycare is close to the center of Anchorage and will be a longer drive, but does have pickup and return service.

Today is Saturday, December 30, 2017. I just informed Pat's son about the change in day care centers. He immediately brought it up in his phone, and I'm sure we'll discuss the change when we go to lunch with him and Pat's daughter tomorrow after church. However, before we meet them for lunch, I'll drive Pat by the daycare facility. This coming Tuesday will be what they call a "trial run," as it will be Pat's first time. And, hopefully, she will like the experience and want to continue. Her schedule will be four days a week (Monday, Tuesday, Wednesday, and Thursday). She will be picked up from our home at approximately 12:30 p.m. and return at approximately 5:00 p.m. The hours of our VA sponsored chore helper have had to be changed because of the totally different daycare hours. Have told Pat about this change, but know that she won't remember, so repetition of this information will be necessary. Probably have to tell her at least six times before next Tuesday.

Today is Wednesday, January 3, 2018. Pat's first day at Hearts and Hands went well. The driver (Alex), who picked her up was very personable, on time, and did have a little difficulty finding our home. He did have two other clients in his vehicle, so Pat sat next to him in the front seat. She did complain to me about "getting rid of her again," but conversed with the driver as they departed. The time of the pickup was about twelve thirty, and the time she was delivered home was 4:30 p.m. Yesterday, her group was delivered to a Value Village store where Pat spent $16 of the $20 I had given her. So the majority of her daycare time was spent on the road going to and from their location and to and from the field trip. Upon arriving home, Pat had no comments about her day, but she did say she really missed me. Upon arriving home, she immediately fixed herself something to eat and drink, and then proceeded to play her computer games.

Monday, January 8, 2018. The weekend went well, with just a couple of times that Pat expressed her anger regarding her dementia. She did lots of walking when we attended a couple of basketball games at the Alaskan Airline Center. A chocolate candy bar and a drink are items that I purchase for Pat after we enter the arena. She will have a seat next to me, but she cannot sit and watch the game. She will walk around the arena and chat with folks as I watch her and the game. She always is able to find her way back to her seat after her walk. During the course of our time there she has to make two or three trips to the restroom, but she has no problem with her restroom visits.

Pat did enjoy our visit to church on Sunday. She handled our communion service well. After the church service, she had no desire to visit and chat with folks, but was anxious to get in our car and head for home. Sunday afternoon we did play Scrabble, a game Pat really enjoys. While I watched sports on TV and did some reading, Pat played her computer games. She was unhappy when I told her we had no plans to leave our home. Upon my insistence, she did take her PM pills, got into her nightgown, and was in bed by 10:30 p.m. She was almost asleep when I joined her about eleven. I had a great night's sleep, but I'm not sure how soundly Pat slept. I was up at 7:30 a.m., and Pat was in bed until 10:30 a.m. Last week, she was pretty determined that she did not want to go to daycare again. This morning, she was okay when I told her that the daycare vehicle would pick her up between 12:30 and 1:15 p.m. I just wished she would give me a report on her daycare experience, but her lack of memory will not make that report possible.

Today is Wednesday, January 10, 2018. We will visit Turnagain Social Club this morning. Back home from our visit and found this very busy center to be one that Pat will enjoy more than Hearts and Hands. We are starting there next Monday, with five-hour-a-day sessions, four days a week. She will be picked up at approximately 11:00 a.m. and be delivered home between 4:30 and 5:00 p.m. The Turnagain Social Club does not offer field trips, so Pat will spend less time in transit and more time doing fun things at the center. I was very impressed with the freedom that Pat will enjoy as she participates.

Chapter 7

*T*oday is Sunday, January 28, 2018. I had a hard time waking Pat up at 9:30 a.m. for our 10:30 a.m. drive to our church located in midtown Anchorage. I still can't understand why nights do not allow her sound and healthy sleep. She's remaining in bed longer and longer, but I don't believe it's quality sleep. She complained to me about her desire to stay home, so we did. However, she was eager to go shopping at Walmart. This was not a good experience for me, as Pat did not remain where she said she would be while I picked up her prescriptions. I must have spent approximately twenty minutes searching the store for her. She had put several items in the shopping cart, most of which we did not need. I was so frustrated with this shopping experience that I left before getting the things on my list. Pat had lost her purse, so I did wait while she replaced the lost lipstick. I had planned to stop at a restaurant, but had wasted so much time looking for Pat, we came directly home after shopping.

I was extremely impressed with Marlow Manor and feel it would be an ideal home for Pat. And possibly myself, at a later date. Talking to Norma Reece today, she felt it would be much sooner for Pat to move into their care facility than if I was to move in at the same time. A larger sized living area would be necessary if I moved in at the same time Pat did. There's a much longer wait for the larger sized units. So now it's a waiting game for Medicaid and for Marlow Manor.

Today is Wednesday, February 7, 2018. Received a call yesterday from Kirsten Smart, a care-coordinator that Norma Reece of Marlow Manor recommended. Kirsten is wondering if the proper procedure has been followed in my pursuit of Medicaid financial help. She's wondering if my care-coordinator has done a plan of care yet. She's also wondering if we've had a visit from Senior Services regarding Pat's level of disability. This phone person would be an employee of the State of Alaska and do a screening of Pat's abilities and a plan of care. She also mentioned that we would receive something called a Denali Card. From talking to Sarah Lawrence a few minutes ago, I found out that the State of Alaska, after the screening phone interview, will send a coupon which will authorize Pat to receive the Medicaid waiver. Before that happens, we will probably have to update Pat's files. The process is long, and the rules are not clear, but I guess the Medicaid waiver will happen and help us to financially handle the cost of the 24/7 care Pat needs. Long-term care monies and Medicaid funds will not happen at the same time. I've been told.

Today is Wednesday, February 14, 2018 (Valentine's Day). I have a phone interview this afternoon at 2:30 p.m. regarding our eligibility for the Medicaid waiver. The phone interview happened as scheduled, and the next step is for the public assistance person to send a coupon to my care-coordinator. Hearing this, I called my care-coordinator and informed her that she would receive a coupon. When she receives the coupon, there will be additional paperwork to be signed and more interviews scheduled. The trail of paperwork is long, and the procedure is very difficult for care-coordinators to understand and explain to those of us trying to find out if Medicaid financial help can become a reality.

Today is Tuesday, February 20, 2018. On Friday, I received four letters from the State of Alaska Long-Term Care team that pertained to my request for the Medicaid waiver. These letters are rather ambiguous. Some of the information requested I've already done several months ago, but will update the information requested. If my care-coordinator is available I need to discuss the information received. May need to find a lawyer to help me obtain the Medicaid waiver. They have denied me my Adult Public Assistance request because I have too much monthly income.

Today is Monday, February 25, 2018. I just got off the phone with the office manager of Marlow Manor. She makes the decision as who is admitted to this 24/7 care facility. In the next few days, they will have available, what they call an alcove living area. This area is between 370 and 385 square feet. They will accept my MetLife long-term insurance and Medicaid if I qualify for the Medicaid waiver. Not sure if they will take our Social Security. I need to ask that question. Once they offer us a unit we have three days to say yes or no. The Alcove unit has 8 × 13 living area, a bedroom area, measuring 12'7" × 10", a kitchen area measuring 9'5" × 12'9" and a bath 5'8" × 6'.

This afternoon, I received a call from Norma Reece, who determines who is admitted to Marlow Manor. She informed me that there is an alcove apartment that will be available on March 10. She would like to know prior to Friday, March 2, if we are going to take the apartment. The cost of this alcove apartment is $6,500 a month.

In arriving at the answer to her question, I have some decisions to make. First, I have to call MetLife representative, Carlyne Russell to find out what monthly amount MetLife long-term care will pay. Then I have to call my care-coordinator, Sarah Lawrence, and find out when we can expect an effective day for Medicaid waiver financial assistance. Will need financial help from both to pay the cost of Pat's care.

Today is Wednesday, February 28. Hard to believe that my phone calls to both Carlyne Russell (MetLife) and Sarah Lawrence (care-coordinator) have not resulted in any response. There's been no reply to my request for help. Since I don't know what financial help I'll receive, I will have to say no to Marlow Manor about moving Pat into their facility. Pat's care will continue to be my responsibility, and her enjoyment of life will be dependent upon the decisions I make. At this time, she continues to ask me each day what fun things I have planned for us. She is not happy when I tell her we are spending a relaxing evening at home. She is constantly asking me to fix dinner for her, however, her food consumption is so minimal that she seldom eats much of what I prepare. Her dementia has caused her to be a grazer, which means we seldom eat a meal together. She is constantly complaining about being hungry, but then finds no appetite after she dishes up food. Her eating, or rather lack of eating, has led to many discussions with her doctors. However, there does not seem to be a pill that helps.

Today is Wednesday, March 6, 2018. Pat has become less argumentative and more docile. She doesn't argue with me, but is more receptive about our plans for fun things and is more than willing to allow me to make all the decisions. She is constantly requesting kisses and forgets that she just kissed me a couple minutes earlier. She is slowly getting her anger under control, and I think she realizes that it upsets me. I have to get rather vocal and let her know that I do not condone her physical reactions when she thinks about the memory destructiveness of her dementia. Her inability to sew, play computer games, read, and focus on television programs result in boredom, and cause her to go to bed, even though it's much too early for sleep. Consequently, she's constantly complaining about being very tired. It is imperative that I insist that she take her before-bedtime pills. She always has to ask me where the pills are located. We always keep them on our kitchen table. The past few nights, she has not wet the bed, although she did have a control problem when we attended her ArtLink class at Alzheimer's. There's bowling tonight, and I know this she really enjoys and does well, although she does have a hard time being available when it's time for her to bowl. She really enjoys walking through the alley area and conversing with her fellow bowlers.

Today is Saturday, March 10, 2018. Pat got up at 10:30 a.m. and went down to the kitchen for coffee and her pills. She then went to her recliner where she was at noon. Checked our bed and found out she did wet it. Nothing was said to me, so while she's snoozing, I have done the laundry. She will be upset when she finds out that I have no plans for fun things today, although I may take her to

Value Village for shopping and then to Olive Garden's for lunch. Because of Pat's extremely small appetite, we will go somewhere where we can make do with one lunch, with me eating over three/fourths of the food we receive. Pat's lunch will be more soda than food. When we get home, she will probably go to the fridge for ice for another soda. She is always thirsty and constantly having a soda. At this time, it's usually root beer.

Have learned this week that Pat and I will be put on the active list for the Palmer VA Pioneer Home, but only after they receive our medical history from the VA. According to the VA, our medical histories have been sent, but the VA does not know where they are.

The really big question that I need answered is, when are we going to find out about our request for Medicaid waiver insurance? I have been attempting, through my care-coordinator, to find out the answer to this all-important question. The paperwork is unbelievable and nobody seems to know how this program works, and supposedly, nobody cares. It has been fourteen months since I initiated my request for help, and I still don't have an answer. If there is no Medicaid waiver help, I will not be able to afford the cost of care for my wife and myself. Being eighty-two years of age with a few health problems, care of my seventy-nine-year-old wife, who is suffering from Alzheimer's, will be next to impossible. Being a tax-paying resident of Alaska for fifty-eight years, I feel I need and deserve some help in my present predicament.

Today is Saturday, March 17, 2018. This past week, I sent a letter to Senator Lisa Murkowski regarding our desperate need for Medicaid waiver insurance. Which is necessary for our move into a 24/7 care facility. Received a call back from her office that they had forwarded my letter to Gov. Walker. Now I'm waiting to hear from his office.

Pat is definitely losing her enthusiasm for life and her desire to do fun activities. When not going to her four-day-a-week daycare, she spends much of her time at home either in bed or in her recliner. Yesterday, she soaked her clothes with urine while in bed and while sitting in her recliner. Her bladder control has left her, and she does not inform me of the need to clean up after she has peed. When she gets up this morning, I will request that she take a shower. I can't be too demanding, but I have to just mention that there's a need for her to shower. Demands make her extremely angry.

Chapter 8

*T*oday is Monday, March 19, 2018. Yesterday, Pat spent most of the day sleeping in her recliner. She didn't get up until one thirty in the afternoon. She was exceptionally quiet, and had little interest in eating or conversing. She just wanted to try and sleep the whole day through. I was concerned about her, and finally talked her into playing Scrabble with me. After our game, she went back to napping in her recliner. She did ask me what we were going to do later in the evening. This she asks me every day—actually, several times during the day. No memory leads to duplication of questions all day long. Late in the day, I decided to move to our second floor and do some writing, using our computer. About 8:00 p.m., I decided to go downstairs and check on Pat. Was real surprised when I didn't find her in her recliner. Found her in our bedroom. Thought it was much too early for bed. Asked her if she had taken her before-bed pills, which she said she had. However, upon checking, I found that she had not taken her pills. So I took the pills and some water to her bedside and watched her take both pills and water. I was quite concerned that there was no kiss before bed, nor were there any words said about her need for sleep.

Yippee-skippy! She did not wet the bed last night! However, I had an extremely difficult time getting her up this morning. She mumbled that she just wanted to stay in the coziness of her warm bed. I had to get her up earlier than usual as she had a 9:00 a.m. appointment with her VA doctor. She wasn't happy about the thought of seeing her doctor. There was nothing of her usual smile, but instead, her facial expression was one of, "Be careful of what you say or…" I can read her facial expression and know when to say nothing. Words will only aggravate the situation. We had a shorter than usual wait for the doctor, but Pat still complained. Dr. Grant took one look at Pat and instantly knew that she was not a happy patient. The doctor had questions for me and pretty much ignored Pat. I explained that Pat did not wear her hearing aids, so conversation with her was pretty difficult. I'm not sure why Pat has such a difficult time wearing both her hearing aids and her dentures. When she takes them out, she never leaves them in the same place, so I spend much time doing a search. There are appointed places on the kitchen table for both, but Pat's dementia doesn't allow her to remember these places. The doctor did write a prescription for some pills that would help with Pat's lack of appetite, and did authorize the VA to send us night diapers, and urine absorption pads for our bed. She is going to complete the required paper necessary for Pat to be admitted to the Palmer VA Pioneer Home. Also, the doctor authorized a chest x-ray and another blood test. Was surprised when Pat was agreeable to have both done, although she said she was both tired and hungry. She was quite unhappy when I dropped her off at the daycare center. I thought it was a very productive day and was very thankful for the doctor's help. Later in the morning, I was helped by a care-coordinator at the Alzheimer's center.

Today is Wednesday, March 21, 2018. This is the day Pat and I go bowling. She will be extremely happy to hear this, as she does love bowling. I just have to make certain she's close to the alley when it's her time to bowl. With all the tiredness she's experiencing lately, I'm sure she'll be ready to leave after the first game. Three games are just too much, but she's game to continue, but she just complains.

I received a call from my care-coordinator this afternoon. It sounds like we're getting closer to the interview that will enable us to get the funds we need from the Medicaid waiver program for Pat's care at the Alaska Veterans & Pioneers Home care facility. We're just waiting for a call from the Medicaid people regarding the level of care Pat needs.

Today is Saturday, March 24, 2018. Pat and I went to a funeral yesterday for the spouse of a lady who attends our Alzheimer's caregivers' group. It was a rather long service, and I was glad that Pat handled it well, even though she couldn't understand. Don't think she understood what this service was all about. Her only comment was about the size of the worship area where the service was held. She expressed a need for food after the service, but she didn't complain when I drove directly home. Use of a bathroom was a necessity for me.

Once home, Pat immediately asked me what we were doing later. She had no comment when I told her we were spending the rest of the day and evening enjoying our home. After filling her glass with root beer, she settled in her recliner for an afternoon snooze, while I watched the NCAA basketball tournament games on TV. Fixed her a hamburger sandwich for supper, but she had little appetite, so most of it went into the garbage. She is now taking some prescription medicine that Dr. Grant recommended for her lack of appetite. Her lack of memory will not allow her to remember her need for the eight pills and some liquid medication that are sitting on our kitchen table. It's my job to remind her and to watch her take her medication each morning and before bed. It's impossible to measure the effectiveness of all the prescribed medicine.

Church yesterday, was followed by lunch with Pat's daughter and son-in-law at Applebee's. Pat had a couple glasses of soda and a couple of tablespoons of her French onion soup. I hated to see the soup returned for disposal. Our Sunday afternoon was spent doing our favorite things. I read, wrote, and had a long phone conversation with a good friend and watched an NCAA basketball game, while Pat spent the afternoon in her recliner sleeping. Late in the afternoon, Pat decided to get her pajamas on. As she left the recliner, I noticed she had wet her pants. Before Pat changed into her nightgown, I smelled something cooking, and asked Pat the cause of the smell. I got up immediately and discovered that Pat had turned on a burner sometime earlier. The blazing burner was in the process of destroying an empty pan, and at the same time had set off our smoke detector. Pat gave me a blank look, and at the same time dropped same pasta noodles in the scorched pan. I couldn't believe her behavior and realized that she had no feelings about a tragedy she could have caused. I now realize that I cannot leave her alone and need to be aware of her every move. I worry about her time spent at the daycare center. I'm sure they are well aware of what problems dementia folks can cause, and how they need supervision.

Today is Tuesday, March 27, 2018. A worker at the Turnagain Social Club called me this morning and informed me of the growth on Pat's eyelid. She said that Kori felt that it should be checked out by a doctor. I've called Pat's VA doctor, and the earliest I could get her in is Tuesday, the third of April. So next week, Pat will see doctors on Tuesday, Wednesday, and Thursday. She really dislikes doctor's visits, especially the waiting. Dementia has caused a lack of patience.

Wednesday, March 28. Yesterday I called the Palmer VA Pioneer Home and left a message regarding Pat's health history paperwork. Earlier, I had been told that it had been faxed to the Pioneer Home headquarters in Juneau. However, the Juneau Pioneer Home Senior Services Technician, Nicole Fenumiai, said that it has not been received, nor had it been received by the Palmer VA Pioneer Home. I am now waiting to hear from someone on Pat's primary care doctors team as to the destination of this important paperwork.

Saturday, March 31, 2018. Good news this past week! While Pat was in her ArtLink class at Alzheimer's, a care-coordinator informed me that we will have a meeting in our home on Thursday morning at 10:00 a.m. with our care-coordinator and a representative of Medicaid. We will be answering questions regarding the level of care Pat needs, which will determine how much financial help we will receive from the Medicaid waiver program. Hopefully, the amount of the financial help we receive will pay for most of the cost of the 24/7 care.

Friday, April 6, 2018. Yesterday, we had our morning meeting with a lady from the Medicaid waiver program.

This meeting, which was held in our home, was attended by our care-coordinator, Pat's son, and my son-in-law. Because of a computer glitch, the scheduled Medicaid representative did not arrive until 11:00 a.m. She spent approximately an hour and a half quizzing my wife and myself. Because of my wife's dementia and inability to remember, many questions had to be answered by myself. At the end of this question-and-answer session, I was told that it would be approximately a month before a decision regarding my wife's eligibility for Medicaid waiver financial assistance would be reached. My assessment of this meeting was that many questions asked were unnecessary, and that the Medicaid person doing the questioning should have the ability to make the determination as to the verdict regarding our request for financial care monies.

The necessary paperwork has been completed that will allow my wife to be put on the active list for admittance to the VA Pioneer Home located in Palmer, Alaska. Also, I have completed the admittance paperwork for the Providence Horizon House 24/7 care. This facility is located in Anchorage. If they will accept Pat, then I will put in the necessary paperwork for me to live there with Pat. Pat and I wait for both the Medicaid waiver approval and an acceptance to live either in the VA Pioneer Home in Palmer or the Providence Horizon Home in Anchorage.

Today is Wednesday, April 11, 2018. I received a call this morning from Adriana Shipowick, social worker at the Palmer VA Pioneer Home. She informed me that Pat had been put back on the active list, but could not tell me when there would be a room for her. As for me, she thought they had received the necessary paperwork, but so far, they have not put me on the active list. So we cannot make any moving plans until the light turns green.

Sharing, what I have seen happen to my wife, as she walks down this road of life's darkest disease, may help others who are a caregiver of a friend or family member who is going to walk this same terrible road.

Today is Tuesday, April 17, 2018. I heard from our care-coordinator yesterday and was informed that Pat is eligible for Medicaid waiver financial help. So I now need to find a place for her that will accept her and accept Medicaid waiver money and long-term care money. So far the three places I have contacted are the VA Pioneer Home in Palmer, Providence Horizon House, and Marlow Manor. At this time these three homes have no space for her, but have her name on their list. I have filled out all the necessary paperwork for all three locations.

Today is Saturday, April 21, 2018. This week has been quite interesting. A letter from the Medicaid people indicate that the final hurdle before Pat qualifies for the Medicaid waiver financial assistance is the approval from the Division of Disabilities Services. This approval is necessary before she can receive home and community-based services. Our care-coordinator is working on getting this approval. I did receive a several-page report on the results of the assessment that we had with the person who represented the Medicaid waiver folks. This report came from Cindy Leong, Senior Services, CAT Intake and Assessment Unit, State of Alaska Department of Health and Social Services. Based on this information, we're almost to the point where we'll get the financial help we need to put Pat in a care facility.

Early this last week, I made a visit to Campbell Creek House and was greatly impressed. Not only with the home itself, but with Sandy Vasquez, the lady who had the home built three years ago, and who oversees the operation. She gave me a tour and the required admittance paperwork for both Pat and myself. Have filled out Pat's paperwork and returned it to Sandy. Now I'm working on my admittance paperwork and plan to submit it sometime this next week.

Think I can now see light at the end of this long tunnel into dementia darkness. By the light at the end of the tunnel, I'm referring to the dark tunnel created by the lack of clear information regarding the sequence of paperwork and interviews necessary to obtain the Medicaid waiver benefits. It has taken me eighteen months to walk through this dark tunnel. Tomorrow at 11:00 a.m., Sandy Vasquez and her nurse will come to our home and determine what level of care Pat needs when she moves into their care-facility.

Tuesday, April 24. Their visit yesterday was rather eye-opening, and what was to have been a half hour visit turned into an hour and a half. The nurse (Christine) quizzed Pat extensively about what she could do and what she couldn't do, while I discussed with Sandy the details involved in getting Pat admitted. Because of Pat's dementia, I was constantly asked to substantiate Pat's answers, while at the same time, sharing information with Sandy. Pat was not her usual talkative self and sat quietly trying to both hear and understand the questions. Pat had no comprehension as to what this meeting was all about. When her questioning was completed, she closed her eyes and tried to sleep. After it was decided that Pat could move into the Campbell Creek House on the first of May, I presented both Sandy and Christine with the writing I had done about Pat's walk into dementia. I also gave them the paperwork from her Medicaid questioner, and my admittance paperwork. I had forty-eight pages of descriptive writing concerning Pat's dementia demise. I also gave Sandy information paperwork about my MetLife long-term care coverage. Our meeting ended with a walk-through of our home.

This morning, I have made several phone calls asking for guidance regarding the decision about selling or renting our home. Before these phone calls, I asked for divine guidance. The first call was made to my son, Dan. The second call was made to a good friend (Bob). The third call came from Pat's son (Bob), and the fourth call was to Sandy, the admittance lady at Campbell Creek House. I also made a fifth call to a real estate agent, Terry Beal. Terry said he will look up particulars on our home and call me later today to make an appointment time for his visit. The consensus of these calls was that renting the house might be best. However, I want to wait for Terry's input before making this major decision.

Pat had not only wet the bed, but had added bowel movement to her mess. I asked her to take a shower immediately after getting out of bed, but she went directly to the kitchen table and had coffee and glanced at the paper. I had to physically help her remove her wet and bowel-movement-filled clothes, and then had to clean up the bathtub after her shower. Ended up throwing out her pants that were filled with bowel movement. Had to clean off the coins that were shit-covered. I was able to get her cleaned up and ready for the daycare driver. Did send extra pants with the driver.

She was transferred to our home by the daycare driver at approximately 4:30 p.m. She then went to our kitchen for a look into the fridge for ice cubes for her soda drink. Then she sat at the kitchen table, sipping her drink and watching the windstorm we were experiencing. I tried to get her to tell me about her day at daycare, but she had no comment. After sitting quietly at the table watching the trees doing strong, wind-blown dances, she moved to her recliner for an attempt at sleep. While she was sleeping, I watched a couple hours of news, and fixed myself a hot roast-beef sandwich. After that, I took the clothes out of the dryer and started making our bed. Pat did come up to help me, but left me as she decided she was in the way. She went to the computer for computer games, where she is right now. I'm leaving to go down and watch *Dateline*.

Wednesday, April 25. Guess the most important phone call yesterday was from our two care-coordinators. In a three-person phone call they told me that they would do the final paperwork required by the Medicaid Waiver decision makers. This paperwork, when signed by all parties concerned, will allow us to receive the Medicaid waiver monies necessary for Pat to move into the Campbell Creek House. This will be her new permanent home, and allow her to receive the care she desperately needs. At this point, I'm not sure how I'll handle my situation. I may eventually move into the same care facility to be near her. I probably won't qualify for Medicaid as I do have assets that need to be moved into a trust before the Medicaid waiver can financially support my care.

Today is Thursday, April 26, 2018. After a very tough day with Pat, I was tired, and went to bed an hour and a half earlier than usual. When I left for bed, Pat was playing games on her computer, which is located right next to the bedroom. She told me she would be right in after she played a little longer. I slept really hard until about 2:00 a.m. Woke up to find that Pat was not in bed and not at her computer. Was surprised to find her sound asleep in her recliner, located downstairs near our kitchen. She seemed to be sleeping peacefully, so I didn't disturb her. Seven in the morning was breakfast for me, and Pat slept right through my breakfast-making. I had a very difficult time getting her up for her 11:00 a.m.

Today is Saturday, April 28, 2018. Yesterday, during Pat's Art-link class, I signed all the necessary paperwork that will allow the Medicaid waiver insurance to happen. The Medicaid wavier insurance is essential for the cost of Pat's care, and should happen within two or three weeks. Once the level of care is approved, the Medicaid money for Pat's daily twenty-four-hour care will happen. Space for Pat is available now at Campbell Creek House. However, I will have to pay $7,200 a month for her until the day that the Medicaid waiver is officially in effect. Not knowing that official date, I wonder about the wisdom of putting and paying for Pat's care next week. I'm supposed to sign a contract for her care at the Campbell Creek House this next Monday or Tuesday and have her move in. The $205 a day charge starts when she is in her new home. At this time, I'm thinking of postponing contract signing until I know for sure that the Medicaid waiver is happening and will pay the cost of care. I'm very capable of caring for her during the waiting period. However, I do realize that Medicaid waiver will not happen until Pat is in a care facility, so I may be forced to put her in and then pay the daily $205 until Medicaid waiver happens. Facing the challenges of obtaining Medicaid waiver has caused me to wonder if the end result is worth the frustration and mental strain.

When explaining my Medicaid predicament to my son, Dan, and his wife, Erin Bashaw, I was told by Erin to contact MetLife long-term care and ask them to cover the daily Campbell Creek House charges that will need to be paid at the time that Pat gets her room. I will definitely make this call on Monday morning, April 30. With the help of family, we will get Pat moved on Tuesday, May 1.

Wednesday, May 2, 2018. This morning, I was finally able to make contact with our MetLife long-term care representative. She is going to get the paperwork necessary for MetLife to reimburse us for expenses that will not be paid by Medicaid waiver. Guess it will be sixty to ninety days before we can submit invoices.

Thursday, May 3, 2018. I had planned to move Pat into the Campbell Creek House on Saturday, but the director of admissions has requested that I wait until Monday, May 7. Hopefully, Pat's son Bob will be back from a Seattle weekend trip and will be available to help with this move. If not, I can do what needs to be done without help.

Saturday, May 5, 2018. I asked the woman who helps with our home problems to work today. Her name is Josefina. She is paid by Compass, and Compass is contracted by the VA. Once Pat is moved into Campbell Creek House, financial help from the VA will be for her VA doctors and the Campbell Creek care.

Monday, May 7, 2018. It's a very sad day in both Pat's life and mine as she moves into her new home on Chester Creek. This day is the beginning of the final chapter in our lives. She has been the love of my life, and I've been the love of her life. The darkness of dementia has not destroyed that love, but has made it stronger for me, while Pat has walked into a world of fuzziness which has caused her to lose feelings that were once so prevalent. Dementia has destroyed her ability to have and express feelings of love and caring. Her new world will be one of confinement, loss of freedom, and a total dependence on the care given by those at the Campbell Creek House. I only hope she will accept the huge changes in her life without aggression and self-destructiveness. I will always love her, even as we lose our physical togetherness. Today, her daycare driver will pick her up as usual, but he will not bring her home after daycare, but will transport her to her new home at the Campbell Creek House.

Chapter 9

*T*oday is Tuesday, May 8, 2018. Yesterday, I took quite a load of things for Pat's new home. Was there to greet her when she got off the station wagon that brought her from the Turnagain Social Club. She was very angry when I again explained to her that Campbell Creek House was going to be her new home. She had no interest in the things in her room, but complained of being hungry and wanting to go to our home on Our Road. She was just plain mad about everything and accused me of getting rid of her. Explaining was futile. While she laid on her hospital bed, I continued to organize her much-too-small room. She had no interest in helping, but constantly complained about everything.

About five thirty, my daughter, Susan Berger, came to help organize her room, and later Pat's son and daughter came to visit with her. No amount of visiting would lessen her desire to leave, nor her anger at being placed in this home. About six, the staff asked all of us to leave so they could help Pat in her adjustment to her new surroundings. I left with an extremely heavy heart and shed some tears on my way home. To handle my sorrow at moving Pat, I did laundry, made the bed, tried to watch television, and made myself a huge chocolate milkshake. I found my thoughts were on Pat, so television watching was impossible. I ended up listening to music and telling myself that everything would work out for both Pat and myself. I went to bed early, and thoughts of Pat were replaced by heavy sleep. It had been an extremely emotional day and one that I hope never happens again.

Yesterday, I found out from Sandy, the supervisor at Campbell Creek House, that after I left on Monday, Pat had been impossible to control. She would not stay in her room, became very belligerent, and roamed the facility, stopping in various rooms to attempt sleep. She urinated in the beds in these rooms, causing the night staff much clean-up. Sandy said her behavior caused much fear to both staff and patients. Finally, at 4:30 a.m., they were able to get her into her own bed and to sleep. Hearing about her bad behavior, I realized I would have to play a bigger part in helping her handle her new change in lifestyle. The road into dementia is getting pretty rough.

Yesterday, at about 3:00 p.m. I went to see her as she arrived from the Turnagain Social Club daycare. Her excitement in seeing me was short-lived, as she was more concerned about going to our hillside home and her two cats. She will not accept the fact that she has dementia and the care she needs is at the Campbell Creek House which is now her new home. Her zest for living is still there, but not at the same level that it was before dementia.

Friday, May 11, 2018. Yesterday was spent with Pat from 3:00 p.m. until I returned home at approximately 11:00 p.m. During my time with her at the Campbell Creek House, we went for a long walk on the bike trail located adjacent to the home. It was a very nice sunny day, and it's really a nice, forest-covered area. We probably walked too far, as we both became extremely tired. From Pat's questions, as we returned to the Campbell House, I realized that she would have been easily lost if I hadn't been with her. Not only lost outside of the Campbell Creek House, but she's unable to find her room without help. Her three attempts to leave the confines of the house by herself resulted in the home's administrator, Sandy Vasquez, returning her back to her room, and informing me as to her attempt to escape. After hearing this, I decided it was time to break our contract and take her back to our home. In retrospect, I think this is exactly what Pat hoped would happen. I requested her medication, before driving a very quiet Pat back to our home. It had been an extremely tough four days and nights at the Campbell Creek House. Their failure to handle her made me realize that there was some tough sledding ahead for both of us.

Once home, Pat's first stop was the fridge for something cold to drink, then the pantry for M&M's, followed by a time spent in her recliner. She had no interest in watching the news but did ask for the TV volume to be turned up. She did ask, "What's for dinner?" Spaghetti, that I had made the previous day was warmed up, but very little eaten. The rest of the day was spent in her recliner searching for sleep. A bowl of ice cream was eaten about halfway through the evening. Before eating ice cream, she said that she needed a root beer, and she became very angry when I told her no. Because of her lack of bladder control, soda just before bed will result in bedwetting. I think she finally realizes that cutting back on liquids three hours before bedtime is necessary.

Today is Monday, May 14. Yesterday, I had planned to take Pat to church; however, because of soreness in her lower back area, she requested we stay home. Later, we went out to lunch with some of her family, before using my truck to transport the things taken to her short-lived Campbell Creek home back to our home. She expressed no visible emotion about returning to our home, and she had nothing to say about leaving the Campbell Creek House. Dementia, besides destroying her memory, has been responsible for an I-don't-care attitude. Have often wondered why she has shed no tears about being a victim of this disease. More anger than sadness is expressed.

Today is Wednesday, May 16, 2018. Yesterday, after Pat was picked up for daycare, I was busy with phone calls. One was to Compass regarding the need to receive her in-home helper again. A call to her care-coordinator regarding her Medicaid waiver request, and a call to VA regarding her need to be authorized for in-home care. After these calls I then drove to the Campbell Creek House to pick-up all Pat's medications, and then on to Walmart for a new prescription that Dr. Fisher had phoned in. This latest script was to relax her before bedtime in hopes she would sleep better. It was then home to get her pills organized. I have a plastic box that I set up for one week of pills. It is compartmentalized for both her morning and evening pills. I have to remind her most days to both take her pills, and where they are located.

Today is Saturday, May 19, 2018. Since we have no doctor's appointments, no daycare, and no scheduled happenings, except for a ten o'clock helper coming for a couple hours, we can enjoy our home. I know Pat will have a problem with this as she gets bored easily and always wants to do something or have something planned. Sleeping and eating will be most important today, plus, she will spend much time playing her computer games.

I was quite surprised, when Pat rolled out of bed shortly after 10:00 a.m. without being prodded to get up. I fixed her some toast and poured her coffee. Since Pat's Compass helper was there to help, I decided I would do some much-needed car-washing of our very dirty Pontiac. It was an extremely tough job as there had been no washing during our very messy spring.

After the washing job, I decided I would put the battery back in our camper and see if there was enough charge in the battery to operate all the needed things necessary for good camping. No power from the battery, so I plugged the camper into an outlet located on the outside of the house. Took a while but finally got the heater working, the water pump functional, the fridge operating, and the propane stove to omit blue flames. Now the purchase of a new battery, and I'm ready to enjoy the beautiful parks in Alaska. Tried camping with Pat last year but found her dementia has destroyed her love of camping. I drove to a nearby park, but upon arriving Pat's only interest was to get back to our cozy and very comfortable home. Today, while I was doing these much-needed projects, Pat was enjoying the comfort of her recliner. It is now 3:15 p.m., and Pat has made the recliner her resting place since right after she had coffee and toast this morning. Wondering if the many pills Pat takes are causing this extreme desire for sleep.

Today is Friday, May 25, 2018. There was only blood work and a diagnostic procedure at the VA and JBER hospital this past week. Hardest part of my caregiver role is to get Pat out of bed and into the shower. I find that shower-taking is getting to be very difficult for her. She doesn't want me to be in the bathroom while she takes a shower, and tries to shut the door in my face. But I need to be there and help adjust the water temperature, and have clothes arranged when she steps out of the shower. Also, she needs my help in putting on her clothes. I've always honored her request and desire for privacy, but my help, even in the shower, is an important part of my care-giving job.

Today I asked one of the Art link class workers if Pat was causing any problems in the class. She gave an immediate no, and said she enjoyed Pat's presence. She was well aware of Pat's very short-lived anger and said that it caused no class-control problems and quickly forgotten.

I look closely at Pat and see facial stress and frustration. This has been especially visible in the last few days. I'm angry at what damage this cruel disease has caused and try to remember the Pat before dementia. She was such a pleasant and very loving person.

After the Art link class, we went across the street to a Kentucky Fried Chicken for lunch. I enjoyed a couple pieces of chicken, while Pat enjoyed the mashed potatoes and gravy, and a soda. Because of her lack of appetite, she has no desire to share the chicken and has trouble eating all the little container of mashed potatoes. After the lunch, we stopped at Fred Meyer's for a few groceries. Pat pushes the cart while I select the items. Earlier in her dementia Pat would have loaded many items in the cart. However, in her current stage she's content to follow me, although she did pick up a couple of items and I gave my approval. Her conversation during our shopping was about her desire to get to the comforts of our home and into her recliner. Of course, the companionship of her cat or cats on her lap is very important. She divided the rest of Sunday afternoon and evening between her recliner, playing games on her computer, and many trips to the fridge and pantry for soda and snacks. There was little conversation with me except about the time, temperature, and what she was going to be doing on Monday. As she walked by me to the different areas of our home, I noticed that her pants and shirt were wet with urine. I asked her to change them. She did change her pants but not her shirt.

I plan to speak to Kori Mateaki, the president and administrator of the Turnagain Social Club. This is the day-care-center that Pat attends four days a week. Kori and her staff deal with Pat's problems during her stay, and hopefully they can help me understand how I can help reduce the frequency of Pat's uncontrolled peeing and bowel movements.

Today is Monday, June 4, 2018. Pat's behavior this past week has helped me reach the conclusion that she needs more help than what I'm capable of giving. Consequently, I've spent the week looking into a couple of assisted living homes that would be right for her. I have the admission paperwork for the Providence Extended Care Facility. This facility is a very large series of several individual home-type buildings. Largest part of their admission paperwork are the many pages that have to be filled out by Pat's VA primary care doctor. I also have visited the Hibiscus Assisted Living Home which is a large home with room for five care-needing individuals. The administrator of this home is a hands-on Hawaiian lady who is extremely pleasant and has an extremely beautiful and well-cared-for home. Right now, she has a very nice upstairs room that is available for

Pat. She does need a payment of $6,500 for the first month of Pat's care. I felt this home was rather dark and not much light coming through the windows. And, of course, I still don't know about Medicaid financial help.

This afternoon we will be visiting Pat's VA Dr. Fisher to have an evaluation of Pat's prescriptions. Her doctor's recommendation may determine which care facility we select. Pat's son, Bob, is going to attend Pat's appointment, as he feels that Pat may be over-medicated.

Today is Tuesday, June 5, 2018. Yesterday's appointment with Pat's VA Dr. Fisher proved quite interesting. The bottom line of this visit was that Pat is definitely being over-medicated. Rather than experiencing brief periods of anger, she now is extremely mellow, with an intense desire to sleep most of the time. She is very quiet, and her main concern is time, temperature, and "What's to eat? I'm hungry." Her doctor thought that the drugs Olanzapine and Divalproex were responsible for this change in her attitude, so for the next two weeks, we will see if a reduction in the amount she takes will bring about a change in her behavior. A very close evaluation of her behavior will be necessary to determine which type of assisted living home will be best for Pat. Whichever home we decide upon, I will have to step out of the picture and allow Pat to adjust to a radically new lifestyle. After twenty-six years of being together, this separation will cause both of us to suffer pangs of sadness. Not sure which of us will suffer the most. Probably myself, as I'm the one that has to make this most difficult decision. While dementia limits Pat's ability to understand, she still loves me and separation will cause her to have feelings of desertion. I only hope that she will accept the care of her next home without anger and without thoughts of self-destructiveness.

Today is Wednesday, June 6, 2018. Yesterday, my daughter, her husband, and my granddaughter spent several hours at our home cleaning Pat's dressing room and bagging a large percentage of her huge quantity of unneeded clothes. A really big job, as we prepare for Pat's move to an assisted living home. Pat arrived home about 5:00 p.m. from her daycare and proceeded to the kitchen for a small snack. She then spent the next couple of hours in her recliner trying to doze. She asked me what we were going to have for dinner. I really hadn't given it much thought, and said I would fix something a little later. Pat did not want to wait, so she decided to fix soup. She had trouble opening the can and asked for my help. The metal opening ring had broken off, so I had some trouble too. As she was downing the soup, I fixed myself a burger and green beans. Pat said her soup was much too salty and left the bowl on the table for me to handle. She then went to her recliner for some napping, while I took care of kitchen clean-up.

Today is Saturday, June 9, 2018. Thursday, this past week was the wonderful day! All my work for the past eighteen months has finally resulted in the care that Pat really needs. Just in time, as the brain destructiveness of the dementia disease has caused her behavior to take a big turn for the worst. In the past month, she has regressed to the point where she will not make any attempt at household chores and expresses anger when asked to take a shower. Her clothes will reek of the odor of urine, but she refuses to change them until I demand she do something.

Thursday morning I received four letters from the State of Alaska, Division of Public Assistance, Long-Term Care Team, informing me that Pat was eligible for Medicaid waiver insurance. Yipee-skippee! Thursday afternoon, I received a call that the VA Pioneer Home in Palmer had rooms available for both Pat and myself. I was really excited about this news and shared it with both my daughter and a good friend who lives in Michigan. The Pioneer Home social worker, Adriana Shipowick, and head nurse, Karen Atherton, told me that I had five days to make a decision as to my acceptance or not. I told them during our phone conversation that I would accept for Pat, but wanted to look over the situation before accepting for myself.

Chapter 10

*T*oday is Sunday, June 10, 2018. I had planned to take Pat to Palmer this afternoon where she would call the VA Pioneer Home her new home, and I would escape the work and frustration of being her caregiver. However, an 8:00 a.m. call from Adriana Shipowick informed me that there was more paperwork before we could move in. More frustration, as the care of Pat is causing my health to deteriorate, and I really feel overburdened by my responsibility. Adriana told me that both Pat and myself needed TB shots. These shots require authorizations from our VA primary care doctors. She also told me that there are eligibility for medical benefits forms to be filled out. She is sending these forms to the Anchorage Pioneer Home, and I will pick them up tomorrow. So the long saga of finding a home for Pat and possibly myself continues.

Today is Thursday, June 14. I was astonished at the amount of paperwork I picked up at the Anchorage Pioneer Home. It took me approximately four hours to get it all filled out. After completing it, I returned it to the Anchorage Home and they will see that it gets to Palmer. Now I'm waiting for Adriana to review and give her approval. Was told by her that we have to be moved in by July 5.

Today is Friday, June 15, 2018. My son, Daniel, turns fifty-six today. A card and some cash went into the mail this morning. Now I'm waiting a return call from Dan as to the handling of our house when Pat and I move into the Palmer VA Pioneer Home. On a previous call from the Palmer Home I did find out that there was a room for me in the independent living area. I decided immediately that I wanted to live there with Pat. More good News!!! Had a message call from Dan about possible renters who had looked our house over a month ago. Guess they are interested.

I've had a touch of the flu the last couple of days, so dealing with Pat's bedwetting and shower needs has been difficult, but I have managed. Took her to her Alzheimer's Art link class this morning. Ten minutes before the class was to end, she was ready to leave for something to eat. She was quite vocal and had no intentions of waiting. But she calmed down when I told her we were going to the VA for TB shots and would eat afterward. At first the shots were not going to happen, but a VA nurse took pity on us, and after she talked to Pat's doctor, they did happen. Guess we won't get the results for a couple of days, but they are necessary for us to move into the home.

When we returned home, there was more good news!! We found three messages on our answering machine. One was from my son, who had been quite surprised to learn of my decision to make the big move. Also, had a message from the admitting social worker at the Palmer Pioneer home wondering if we had our TB shots. The third message was from MetLife about a request I had sent them about a claim for payment on some expenses I had occurred. They will call me Monday about this. These three messages were extremely important, and the resulting conversations will probably determine when we make the big life-changing move to our new Palmer, Alaska, home.

Today is Sunday, June 17. Slept in our upper bedroom last night as Pat forgot which side of the bed she sleeps on, and put herself on the side that I have slept on for many years. So rather than asking her to move, I went to our upper bedroom. Pat does not put on her pajamas or night-gown, but sleeps in the clothes she has worn all day. Her getting-up time yesterday was one thirty in the afternoon, with the rest of her day spent in her recliner. She was back and forth to the fridge and pantry several times for drink, ice cream, and no-bean chili. She complained of being very hungry but had no appetite. When she sees me snacking, she wants the same thing, but eats very little, and I have to throw out what she doesn't eat or put it in the refrigerator.

Today is Tuesday, June 19. Again, Pat was extremely unhappy when I requested that she get her very urine-covered self out of bed and into the shower. It was 9:15 a.m., and we had a ten thirty appointment at her VA doctor's office. It's a good half hour's drive across Anchorage to the Veteran's Administration building. Being very verbal didn't do the get-up job, so I had to remove all her covers along with demanding words. I had put her clothes in our downstairs shower-taking room and had asked our personal attendant helper to be ready to receive Pat and assist her in her shower-taking. This done, I then had to remove her urine-soaked sheets and tuck them into our washing machine. It's a daily ritual in our home.

The really good thing this morning was an 8:00 a.m. call from our MetLife long-term care person informing me that my long-term life insurance would pay Pat's claims from the VA Pioneer Home in Palmer. So glad that the home is now on Metlife's approved list. It had taken many phone calls to get this to happen. Now, if the Pioneer Home admittance person has checked and approved my many pages of paperwork we'll make the huge move this coming Tuesday, June 26, 2018, into our new home. Tomorrow we'll hear the answer to the preceding statement.

Today is Thursday, June 21, 2018. Didn't receive a call from the VA Pioneer Home yesterday as expected, but did get the call this morning. At this time, I need to get the results of our Quantiseron Gold shots into the hands of the Pioneer social worker, Adriana Shipowick. I tried to get the people in the VA Release department to fax the results to Adriana but was told that they can't do that unless I'm there in person to initiate the fax. So I made the half hour drive and caused this transfer to happen. Came home from handling this transfer and found a message from Adriana that she had the results, and that we were free to move in next Tuesday. Excited about this move, but I know that I have a lot of work to do and more paperwork to fill-out to make the big move happen with as little stress as possible.

Today is Saturday, June 23, 2018. I have notified our VA social worker, Compass, Alzheimer's care folks, our care-coordinators, MetLife long-term care coordinator, and family and friends about our Tuesday, June 26, move to the VA Pioneer Home. Most have wished us the best, and family members have volunteered their help. Today, I plan to spend time deciding what we will transfer to Palmer to take care of our immediate needs. I plan to drive the forty-five miles to Palmer as soon as I can get help loading my truck with heavy furniture items. This may happen today, but it will happen for sure on Sunday morning. Pat's son, daughter, and son-in-law, have volunteered to come up to our house at 11:00 a.m. Sunday morning to help load my truck. My recliner, a fairly large table, both TV and radio with stands, small dresser-drawer unit, both computers with printer, and microwave will be on the first truck-load to Palmer. In the back seat of the truck will be our clothes, toiletries, and the wall hangings (a.k.a pictures). If there's room in the bed of the truck, we will include a large bookcase. But this can wait for a later trip.

Today is Sunday, June 24. Our trip to Palmer today was quite successful. With the help of my family and Pat's, we were able to transport heavier items and set them up in our rooms. Found the rooms to be inadequate to hold the furniture we took, but in my room, there is a storage area that will be a temporary home for items I may need later.

Today is Wednesday, June 27, 2018. The last two days have been unbelievable. What a change our life has taken as we've finally made the huge move from living in an eight-room house to two rooms in the beautiful VA Palmer Pioneer Home. It's a bit cramped in my room, and I am planning to take some furniture pieces back to our Anchorage home. Pat's room will suit her needs, as her needs are few. Pat, in her dementia-diseased mind, will not accept the fact that the Pioneer Home is now her home. She is constantly asking me when we are going to our Anchorage home, and gets angry when I explain to her that Palmer is now our home. Hopefully, this move will help both her and me deal with the terrible disease she is experiencing. I understand her thinking, as I still wonder if our big move will be beneficial to both of us. Only time will tell.

Today is Sunday, July 1, 2018. We didn't leave our new VA home yesterday, except when I drove over to a nearby Fred Meyer's store for needed supplies. Surprised, when eating with Pat, that her appetite has definitely improved. So glad to see her eat a good percentage of the healthy meals that they prepare for us. Within a short time after eating, she complains about being hungry. The pangs of hunger are short-lived, as little food is consumed before she says she's full. Pat's desire for food is pretty much continuous all day long. A few of the folks living here are hand-fed by the care-giving employees. The speed of their eating is extremely slow, and the quantity is limited. In the Alzheimer's eating area, there is very little conversation, except between those serving. So sad when one thinks about the reason for their silence.

Today is Tuesday, July 3. The really good news is not about Pat, but about the phone call I received from my son this morning. He called to inform me that a family will rent our home, and that they would like to move in this August. So thankful that it won't sit vacant long. They will make $1,800-a-month payments, plus pay the electricity and the gas bill. With the rental money, it will make it much easier to handle the cost of care for Pat and myself.

Today is Monday, July 9, 2018. Yesterday, Pat's daughter and son-in-law drove up from Anchorage to visit her. They Skyped her daughters who live in the Seattle area. While they were visiting, I was visiting my son, who had just been in a footrace to the top of five-thousand-foot Pioneer Peak mountain. Pat's reactions to our visitors was one of dementia-caused, I-could-care-less attitude. She said little and was more interested in sleep-attempt and eating. I don't believe she verbally told our guests goodbye.

Today is Thursday, July 12, 2018. After observing Pat's behavior since I saw her on Monday, I realized that her walk into the terrible darkness of Alzheimer's has happened. The light at the end of the tunnel has gone out, and the hope that somehow she will return to herself of five years ago is impossible. At this point, I realize that I can do nothing more to help her, and that her existence in this world is coming to an end. How soon I do not know. But I do know that her ability to care for herself is gone and that she is in the hands of care-givers who really care. She has moved into the area of darkness that is occupied by other folks who live and are cared for by the professional care-givers in the Alzheimer's area of the VA Pioneer Home. She will spend her remaining days in this facility.

Today is Saturday, the fourteenth of July. Yesterday was a pretty normal morning for me as I rode my bicycle to get the Anchorage paper, followed by an enjoyable large break-fast. Since Pat's morning was spent in bed, I didn't see her until I went to her area just before the scheduled ice-cream social. When I mentioned ice cream, she was eager to leave her area and join me for this special treat. While we were in my room waiting to enjoy ice cream, a lady knocked on my door. She identified herself as Olga Tanner, our assigned care coordinator from Care Coordination Resource of Alaska. The purpose of her visit was a meet-and-greet session. She was a Medicaid expert and would help us when confronted with Medicaid problems. She did inform me that the Medicaid waiver insurance would cover about 60% of Pat's care expenses while at the Pioneer Home. This news I was especially glad to hear as to date nobody could tell me exactly what Medicaid would pay.

Today is Tuesday, July 17, 2018. Now that my room is organized, I can get Pat's room to look less like a hospital room and more homey. Not that pictures on the walls will mean much to her, but they may be enjoyed by her visitors, if she has any. She's very difficult to communicate with, and mainly concerned with eating and resting, although she does like to walk the hallways of the home and peer into the rooms.

Today, I was informed by one of her nurses that Pat is having a hard time balancing herself due to the strapped flip-flops she is wearing. I've seen that lack of balance myself and suggested that they try to get her to use a walker. The nurse said that Pat told her she did not want to use the walker, but the nurse said she would keep trying to convince Pat that it's necessary to prevent a fall. I know that falling is a real problem with those experiencing Alzheimer's.

I'm having an extremely difficult time deciding how much time I should spend with Pat. Her condition is such that I know she recognizes me, but her need to see me is nothing compared to my need to see her. I think that eventually my need to visit her will decline as I realize my visit will have little effect on her, but is very hard on me, as I view her decline into the dark depths of Alzheimer's. It's a dilemma I have to deal with.

Today is Wednesday, July 18. Yesterday I decided I would spend the day without seeing Pat. It was extremely difficult, as it was against my feeling of obligation. It was a good day, as my mind was centered on happenings here at the home. A friend's invitation to attend a noon luncheon put on by a local Lion's group was enjoyed. Later, I listened to a talented gal play the piano, and late in the afternoon, I listened to my friend Dave sing songs from years past. Pat's always in my thoughts, but found I enjoyed not being responsible for her care.

As for myself, I'm in an independent living area and receive very limited care. After a visit with Pat, I'm depressed as I know I will never see the Pat of years ago. Alzheimer's has taken its toll. I've learned that to ask her questions only cause her confusion and frustration about answering. One or two-word verbal answers are accompanied by a questioning blank look which tells me that I should not have asked such questions.

Because I do not know how Alzheimer's will affect our future, I'm not sure what we will experience in our remaining years. But I do know that this journey is much more difficult for me than it is for her. At this time, her world is the bed in her small room, and a lunchroom which she cannot find without assistance. She is entirely dependent on those caring for her. She is not feeling pain, and is in a very safe environment, and has no problems to solve. Meanwhile, my love for her is everlasting.

As for myself, I've walked into a world I've never, never known! I choose to live here for two reasons. First, and most important, is to comfort Pat and make certain she gets the care she needs. Second, at the age of eighty-three, and watching as my abilities disappear, I may someday need the care provided here. After six weeks of living here, a finer assisted living home I could not have found. The mission of the Palmer VA Pioneer Home is to provide the best care possible for all of its residents. I feel so fortunate that Pat and I are the recipients of this care.

The writing of this story has taken over three years and has given me an insight into a world I did not know existed. I find, that when mentioning Alzheimer's to folks who have not had contact with someone needing the care necessary for survival, I receive a rather blank look. This is understandable, as it's only by being a twenty-four-hour a day caregiver for a person suffering the debilitating effects of this terrible disease can one become aware of the life-changing effects of this disease. It's heartbreaking to watch as one's partner loses her brain-centered abilities.

The keyword, when being a caregiver, is patience. Understanding, would be the second most important word. So to be a good caregiver, patience is absolutely essential, and the need to understand what your patient is experiencing as he or she is victimized by the disease is so important.

As I bring this story to an end, I will mention that fifteen minutes ago I was able, with the help of Pat's personal care helper, move Pat from my bed to her walker, where she very slowly went through the door and into the area where Alzheimer's folks are served their food. Four of the ten Alzheimer's patients in this room need to be hand-fed, each by one of the four personal care attendants. From eating in this area many times, I have found that there is practically no conversation between Alzheimer's patients, but much conversation between the four caregivers.

Hope I have provided food for thought to those in the shoes of a caregiver. A caregiver who's caring for a person whose experiencing life's darkest disease, Alzheimer's.

Today is Saturday, September 27, 2018. As I look back on this writing, I discover that the last date I mentioned was July 18. Pat's life has been pretty much the same each day. Her personal caregiver gets her up each day at approximately 8:00 a.m. After her personal hygiene is handled by the care worker, she is escorted down the beautifully decorated hall to the dining area where she is served food that has been pureed. The puree process is necessary because she will not wear her dentures.

The 8:30 a.m. breakfast is followed by 11:30 a.m. lunch which is followed by 4:30 p.m. dinner. In between meals, she either is taken to her room, watches television in a room that is visited by other Alzheimer's patients, or she is helped into a chair or couch located in the hallway. Since Pat's ability to walk without the possibility of a fall, means that someone has to be by her side as she uses her walker. In the last couple of days it has been decided that she needs to travel by wheelchair. Of course, a wheelchair doesn't allow her the walking exercise she needs. I know that Pat feels that this type of daily living is pretty boring. Fortunately, her lack of memory does not allow her to remember what happened the previous day or the previous hour. She lives for each moment, with little memory of the past and little thought as to her future.

To make her life less boring, I have accompanied her on special bus excursions that the Pioneer Home offers. Their specially designed small buses have lifts that lift wheelchairs into the bus. For safety, each wheelchair is secured with special straps. On excursions, they've taken us to Hatcher Pass and the Alaska State Fair. Pat and I enjoyed both trips.

In the past two weeks Pat has experienced three falls. One fall resulted in a broken wrist and the other one resulted from an infected toe and leg. Each caused me to take Pat to the ER in the nearby Mat-Su Regional Hospital. Just a few minutes ago, I was informed that Pat had fallen again, but no injury. Falls are something that Pat has to learn to avoid.

I've finished this story and hopeful that those reading this will develop a better understanding of this terrible disease. My story ended a few minutes ago. Only God knows how long Pat will have to endure the walk through this dark tunnel of disease.

Please contribute to the Alzheimer's research organization as they attempt to find a cure.

Addendum to "Life's Darkest Disease"

After looking at the year-long plus publishing time, I realize a addendum (addition) is necessary to give readers an up-to-date finish to my story. If the publishing time continues to lengthen, I may be printing my wife's obit as the ending story.

Today's date is September twenty-fifth, 2019. I signed the publishing contract on September twenty-fifth, 2018. I was told by the Christian Faith Publishing Representative that the publishing time process would be 6 to 9 months. It's now a year, and I do not know how much longer before I see the finished book. I have done the final editing, and submitted all the paperwork necessary for Page Design. Now I'm waiting for the editor's to do their job of Page Design. They have given me no completion date for this phase, and will forward Page Design changes for my approval.

As the time of waiting increases, my wife's Alzheimer's experience changes. I cannot control the publishing process, but I can write a addendum covering the changes I've seen in my wife during the year-long publishing process.

Fortunately, my job as Pat's primary caregiver, ended when we entered the Pioneer Home. My primary responsibility, as her husband, is to make certain she receives the care that allows her final days be free of pain, free of anger, free of injury, and that she enjoys a level of living that gives her hope and a little happiness.

The story of the past year is better that I had ever expected.

Her falls, which I mentioned in the last chapter, resulted in the staff telling me that they were going to transfer her from the walker to a wheelchair. I was agreeable, as I knew her walking ability had come to an end. The first nine months of our 15 month stay here were pretty uneventful. I spent a lot of time using a wheelchair to accompany Pat as she maneuvered the hallways. Using a wheelchair, I was down at Pat's level of communication, and able to keep her out of other resident rooms. During this time she was eating well, and accepting the care the personal care attendants were providing. Despite Pat's demands to be taken home, she seemed to be adapting to life in this home.

Recoveries from her falls happened. Although, the healing from her broken wrist and infected toe and leg was somewhat painful and slow, Pat never complained. She was a real trouper!!

Last April, without warning, she lost her color, became despondent, and only wanted to sleep. She had no desire nor energy to wheelchair, and just wanted to stay in her room. A lift had to be used to get her from her bed and her wheelchair. Have many photos of her as she was experiencing this downturn in her life of Alzheimer's. Folks caring for her couldn't believe this change. Really scared me, as I felt her time on this earth was rapidly coming to an end. David Brown, who has lost his wife to Alzheimer's and I visited a Valley Funeral Home & Crematory, where I filled out the paperwork for Pat's cremation and death certificates. I will pay approximately $1,600 at the time I call "Valley Funeral Home & Crematory" and inform them of Pat's passing.

Due to Pat's bad condition, her Pioneer Home doctor, Steve Parker, along with his medical staff, decided to add Hospice (end of life care) to her medical care. Her Hospice doctor is Jeffrey Melendez. I was informed of their decision and asked to sign the necessary paperwork. A Hospice nurse was the assigned to Pat. This nurse pays weekly visits and is responsible for Pat's medication. Her medication is mixed in with the pureed food she eats.

Approximately two months ago there was a huge change in Pat's condition. A change that caught myself and her staff by complete surprise. At night, Pat appeared to be near death, and the next morning a huge change happened. She became very talkative. To the point of being argumentative. Suddenly, she no longer wanted the security of her bed. Her eyes brightened, and her desire to "do something" became prominent in her mind. What a fantastic change!! A wonderful change that gave us reason for hope!! What was the reason for this change!! Nobody knew!! Not even her doctors. Maybe God, using his infinite power. Ours is not to question, but to appreciate.

Today September 26th, she still has that wonderful conversation ability, and the desire to "keep moving", however, her desire to eat has not returned. Purred food is pushed away after testing, and she is always complaining of being tired. I'll keep her active as she propels her wheelchair through the halls of this beautiful Pioneer Home. But, there's no way I can make her eat. She tells me she wants to keep living, and I tell her she has to eat to live. Don't we all!!!

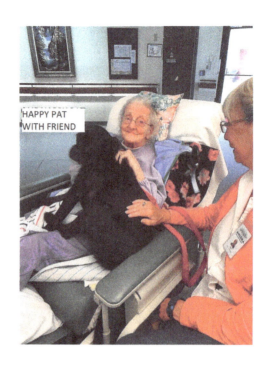

HAPPY PAT
WITH FRIEND

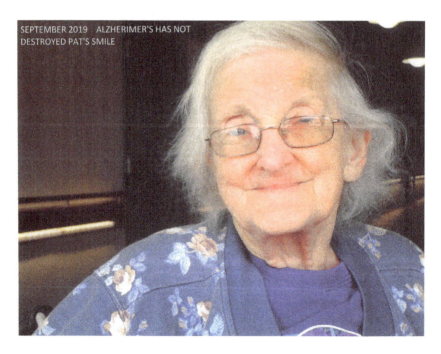

SEPTEMBER 2019   ALZHERIMER'S HAS NOT
DESTROYED PAT'S SMILE

About the Author

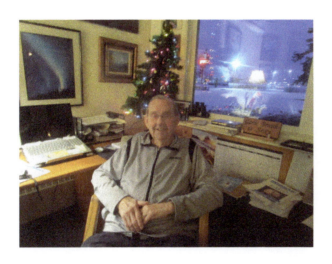

*T*he US Army transported Bill Brokaw to Alaska in 1959. After serving two years, Bill and two military men drove the Alaska Highway to Seattle for separation from the military. After one year of work in Loraine, Ohio, Bill bought a hearse, married, and returned to Alaska. In the last fifty-seven years, he has been involved in managerial work in drug stores, bookstores, and retired from Fed-Ex in 2013.

Before, and during his time in Alaska, he has been very active on the basketball court. At the age of 65, basketball caused a major ankle problem. Rather than give up the sport, he decided to have a new ankle installed. While in the hospital, awaiting ankle surgery, he became a victim of staff infection. This infection destroyed the tissue, and three attempted surgery's kept Bill on crutches for eleven months. Basketball playing over, Bill decided to become a writer. His first attempt was entitled, "Hearse to Hoops". A 1961 trip up the Alcan Highway in a hearse, experiencing the 1964 earthquake, and 40 years of Alaska basketball are shared in his story.

Marriage to his first wife happened in Michigan, before their hearse trip to Alaska. This wife bore him two children. His oldest was conceived in the hearse on the Alaska Highway. He married his second wife in 1992. She entered the world of Alzheimer's four years ago. He has written this story as he observed her suffering from the influence of this terrible disease.

He would like to see his story help others who are caring for a loved-one who is experiencing debilitation caused by this disease.

CPSIA information can be obtained
at www.ICGtesting.com
Printed in the USA
BVHW021454100220
571815BV00006B/8

9 781645 153375